Bach Flower Remedies
for Animals

By the same authors

Stefan Ball

Bach Flower remedies for Men

The Bach Remedies Workbook

Judy Ramsell Howard

The Bach Flower Remedies Step by Step

Bach Flower Remedies for Women

Growing Up with Bach Flower Remedies

Stefan Ball & Judy Ramsell Howard

Bach Flower Remedies for Animals

The definitive guide to treating animals
with the Bach Remedies

Index by Mary Kirkness

Illustrated by Kate Aldous

Vermilion
LONDON

3 5 7 9 10 8 6 4 2

Text © Stefan Ball and Judy Ramsell Howard 1999
Illustrations © Kate Aldous 1999

First published in the United Kingdom in 1999 by
The C. W. Daniel Company Ltd

This edition published in 2005 by Vermilion,
an imprint of Ebury Publishing
Random House UK Ltd.
Random House
20 Vauxhall Bridge Road
London SW1V 2SA

Random House Australia (Pty) Limited
20 Alfred Street, Milsons Point, Sydney,
New South Wales 2061, Australia

Random House New Zealand Limited
18 Poland Road, Glenfield,
Auckland 10, New Zealand

Random House (Pty) Limited, Isle of Houghton,
Corner of Boundary Road & Carse O'Gowrie,
Houghton 2198, South Africa

Random House Publishers India Private Limited,
301 World Trade Tower, Hotel Intercontinental Grand Complex,
Barakhamba Lane, New Delhi, 10 001, India

Random House UK Limited Reg. No. 954009
www.randomhouse.co.uk
Papers used by Vermilion are natural, recyclable products
made from wood grown in sustainable forests.

A CIP catalogue record for this book is available
from the British Library

ISBN: 0091906512
ISBN: 9780091906511 (from Jan 2007)

Designed by Tina Ranft

Printed and bound in Great Britain by William Clowes Ltd, Beccles, Suffolk

For Alexandra, Madeleine & Ethan (SB)

... *for* Sam & Fay (JH)

... and in memory of Christine Newman, who loved
helping animals

Acknowledgements

Many people have helped make this book what it is. At the risk of leaving out the most important we are delighted to acknowledge help received from:

- Heather Simpson, animal behaviourist and registered Bach practitioner, who outlined general principles for us and also gave valuable insights into the legal position of professionals who want to help animals;
- Christopher Day, veterinary surgeon, who also provided information on the legal question;
- the many people who have contacted the Bach Centre by 'phone, fax, letter and e-mail to ask about helping animals – answering these has taught us a great deal;
- the practitioners and members of the public, who have shared their knowledge and experiences with us over a period of years, including in particular Sharon Lloyd, Elaine Hollingsworth and Stefanja Gardener, and the many others whose contributions are acknowledged individually in the text;
- the team at the Bach Centre for their usual unfailing support and good humour;
- our respective partners and children for putting up with the furrowed brows and absent-minded glances that are such an essential part of the creative process;
- and finally, our publishers Ian and Jane Miller at The C.W. Daniel Co. for their limitless patience and elastic deadlines.

Contents

Introduction
Acknowledgements   vi
About this book   ix
About the authors   xi

CHAPTER 1: **The Background**
Historical attitudes: Animals as machines   1
Dr Bach and his discoveries   4
The humanity of animals   8
Do animals have souls?   11

CHAPTER 2: **Using the Remedies**
The role for the remedies   15
The 38 remedies   17
Dosage   39
Legal considerations for practitioners   41
Models for the future   43
Getting the vet on your side   44

CHAPTER 3: **Reading Animal Behaviour**
Principles of selection   46
Verbal communication   49
Non-verbal communication   52
Gender differences   62
Breed differences   63

CHAPTER 4: **Animals in the Home**
Household dogs   67
Dog case studies   73
Household cats   82
Cat case studies   90
Other household animals   101
Small animal case studies   102
Treating the owners   104

CHAPTER 5: **Horses**
    Horse and horse   108
    Horse and rider   113
    Injury and emergencies   118
    From stable to show-ring   120
    Horse case histories   122

CHAPTER 6: **On the Farm and in the Wild**
    Farm animals   125
    Farm case studies   127
    Wild animals   131
    Wild animal case studies   134

CHAPTER 7: **Frequently Asked Questions**   138

CHAPTER 8: **Going on from Here**
    Learning more about the remedies   147
    Learning more about animals   151
    Useful addresses – Bach Flower Remedies   153
    Other useful addresses   154

    Index   156

Introduction

About this book

Dr Bach's work has been used to help animals of all shapes and sizes for as long as the remedies have been in existence. Dr Bach had a dog – a spaniel called Lulu – who received some of his remedies from time to time. His colleague and successor, Nora Weeks, had a series of cats, and they too were all given remedies when they needed them.

The last of them was Wumps, who was most definitely one of the Bach Centre team. He was an independent soul, who liked his morning cuddle but knew how to draw the line. He wasn't one to demand attention or constant petting, but instead was quite happy to wander off on his own to play in the garden to be amused by the bees, butterflies and fish in the pond. Or he would find a warm corner in which to rest and watch the visitors come and go.

Many of these visitors would ask Nora about using the remedies to help their animals, and she would give what help she could. Today out of the hundreds of calls handled at the Bach Centre every week, a good percentage continue to come from people who want to use the remedies to help their animals. So the need for a book to explain how to go about doing this has long been obvious. Indeed, we have been asked time and time again to recommend a reliable book on the subject and have never been able to do so because one didn't exist. In the end we have had to write it ourselves.

Neither author claims to be an expert on animals, but in researching and writing this book we have been fortunate to be able to draw on the generous advice and assistance of many friends, both personal and professional. Practitioners registered with the Dr Edward Bach Foundation, many of whom we have helped train in the remedies, have in turn helped train us in animal lore and have given us the benefit of their experiences. And correspondents around the world have told us stories of how their animal friends have been helped by the remedies.

This book has been a long-cherished project for both of us. We hope that in sharing what we know and what others have shared with us it will make a contribution to the well-being of our fellow creatures, both great and small. If only one animal has an improved quality of life as a result of our efforts, then it will have all been worthwhile.

We hope you enjoy *Bach Flower Remedies for Animals*, and get as much out of the book as we have enjoyed putting in.

About the authors

Stefan Ball got to know the Bach Flower Remedies through his wife, Chris, who trained as a nurse with Judy in the 1970s and started work herself at the Bach Centre in 1991. Occasional odd jobs at the Centre, including translation work and help with educational and audio-visual projects, culminated in a commission to write his first book on Dr Bach and his remedies and an invitation to join the team at the end of 1995, an invitation that he was honoured to accept.

Judy Howard has been working with the Bach Flower Remedies since 1985 when her father John Ramsell invited her to join the team at the Bach Centre, Mount Vernon. John worked with Dr Bach's friends and colleagues, Nora Weeks and Victor Bullen from 1971 and was appointed their partner and successor, so even before she began work at Mount Vernon the remedies were an integral part of Judy's family life.

Judy is a registered nurse, midwife and health visitor, and is a Trustee and Custodian of the Bach Centre. Her husband, Keith, is a keen wildlife gardener and herpetologist, skills which naturally spill over into caring for the garden at Mount Vernon and for the wild creatures who visit it.

CHAPTER 1:

The Background

Historical attitudes: Animals as machines

In the book of Genesis, Adam was given the magical power of naming the animals, so confirming the special position humankind held in relation to the animal kingdom. There was a kind of feudal contract in place, in which humanity's care and responsibility was exchanged for service and fruitfulness. All was balance and harmony in the Garden of Eden.

The story of Noah and the great flood confirmed the ideal of care and compassion for other living things. The animals were not saved simply because they were a valuable resource. They were saved because, like the righteous man Noah and his family, they had intrinsic value as part of Creation. And when the flood was over God made his covenant not just with the human beings, but with all the living creatures who came out of the ark.

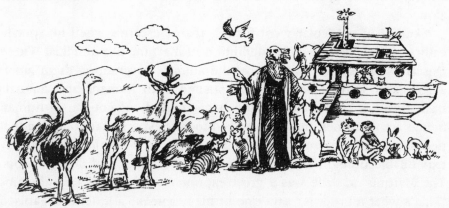

Perhaps that naming ceremony long ago in the book of Genesis was the soil in which our attitudes towards animals, and towards nature in general, first took root. Whether or not this is true, the old feudal ideal of mutual respect and fealty soon withered away as Western philosophy found new ways to understand humanity's place in the natural world.

The new attitude was most famously expressed by the French philosopher René Descartes in the seventeenth century. 'The reason why animals do not speak as we do' he said 'is not that they lack the organs but that they have no thoughts.' Descartes never considered the possibility of non-verbal language. Nor did he consider the emotional bond so familiar to every owner, carer and handler. Animals did not speak, so they must lack both reason and souls. They were just bodies – machines of flesh and blood.

In more modern times this view drew ammunition from the work of the American behaviourist and psychologist Burrhus Frederic Skinner. Skinner, who died in 1990, was very clear that the only possible scientific approach to the study of psychology of animals was to look at behaviour. He gave his name to the 'Skinner box', which was a simple machine used to train rats and pigeons to respond to stimuli. A simple machine to test simple machines: and if animals are machines, without feelings or thoughts or consciousness, and if their only role is to be useful to mankind, then it doesn't really matter what we do with them as long as we make them more useful. The horrors of factory farming and veal crates are a logical result of this point of view.

For a long time animal behaviourists were only interested in studying responses to external stimuli. Anyone claiming to be interested in what animals do spontaneously and of their own accord was a hopeless romantic. Some behaviourists even went so far as to try not to observe animals directly at all, and confined themselves to statistical analysis alone.

Skinner in particular went further than Descartes when he specifically included people in his definition of machine-like animals. Where Descartes raised humanity above the animals by granting them alone a soul and spirit, Skinner firmly pushed both humans and animals back down to the status of mechanism. And, of course, if human beings are machines, there is no need to take especial care of individual people, because seen from a wider point of view they are merely expendable units in an endless series of near identical fleshy robots. The Marquis de Sade was a great exponent of this view of humanity. 'That's what murder is,' says one of his heroines, 'a little disorganised matter, a few changes in the combinations, a few molecules broken up and stuck back into nature's crucible ... where then is the harm in that?'

A few broken molecules, cogs that can be taken apart and allowed to reform, with no particular value attaching to one arrangement rather than another. This is an extreme materialist argument, in which any talk of emotions and common humanity, let alone souls and higher purposes, is redundant and subject only to ridicule. There is nothing higher than this, says Sade, and smashes his machine men and machine women like a disappointed child.

The failure is a failure of imagination and viewpoint. Look, for example, at the computer in your home. A computer at bottom is simply a collection of on-off switches, of ones and zeros, but we all know that computers are far more than this. They can display a picture of the Mona Lisa, flash messages around the world, and simulate the birth of new planets. Fantastically advanced programs are being written that mimic human intelligence, learn from their own experiences and evolve to their own pattern. There are even computers now that can write new computer programs so complex that human programmers find it impossible to follow the logic used.

It would be ridiculous to attempt to describe these activities by writing out a series of ones and zeros. How much more ridiculous it is to describe our loves and ambitions and beauty as the mechanical motion of colliding molecules. Far from being unimportant, as Sade claimed, the arrangement of molecules into complex patterns is **the most important thing there is**. The reality of life is concealed rather than explained by looking at it in mechanical terms.

It should be obvious that animals, like people, are more than the sum of their moving parts. They are intelligent beings, capable of learning by themselves – as squirrels have shown when researchers oblige them to tackle the most intricate obstacle courses in order to reach a dish of peanuts. The way the squirrel works out how to overcome each obstacle is a tremendous display of problem solving ability, which clearly requires thought, memory and intelligence.

If animals are capable of intelligent thought and do not solely rely on instinct to survive, then it is no step at all to assume that they must also have the capacity to feel emotions; and not only that, but also have individual characters of their own. And if they possess these things then we in our turn possess a system of medicine that can help them just as it can help us: the Bach Flower Remedies.

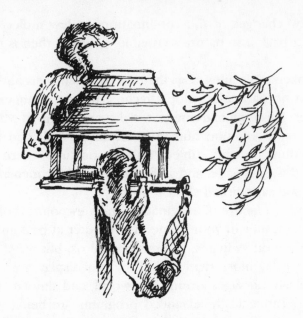

Dr Bach and his discoveries

In 1912, Edward Bach qualified as a medical doctor. It was the fulfilment of a long-held ambition. Ever since he was a child Bach had wanted to be a doctor, or at least to be in a position where he could do something towards the relief of sickness and suffering.

Already, observation of the men working at his father's brass foundry had convinced him that mental attitude had a profound effect on the body, so it was natural that throughout his medical career he would make an active study of human nature. He would sit for hours by his patients' bedsides, listening to them, finding out what manner of people they were, what worried them, what frightened them, how hopeful they were of recovery. He found that patients who had a positive outlook had a better prognosis and got well quicker than those who had a negative perspective of life. And this link between mind, body and spirit, and the conclusion that emotional harmony gives rise to physical well-being, was to form the foundation upon which Dr Bach built his life's work.

Dr Bach's career led him to the study of immunology and to the development of a new group of vaccines that generated a great deal of interest and excitement among his contemporaries. The vaccines had a profound effect on a variety of chronic conditions and the work he did in this area was a major breakthrough in medical science.

Despite his success, Dr Bach was neither happy with the dosage methods he was using – which involved the use of hypodermic needles – nor with the products themselves: intestinal bacteria formed the basis of the vaccines. For this reason he continued his researches in the hope of finding a less invasive method of achieving the same results. He began working with homoeopathy, and on reading *The Organon* by Samuel Hahnemann he felt he might at last have found what he was seeking. Hahnemann's philosophy of treating the patient rather than the disease, and thus the cause rather than the effect, was entirely in accord with his own way of thinking. The homoeopathic principle of the minimum dose, the idea of preparing medicines so that no poison was left, and the method of oral administration which caused the patient no pain, all fitted well with the principles that his own research was leading him to adopt. Thus inspired, he began to make homoeo-pathic preparations of the vaccines he had been working on, and was conscious of having taken a huge step towards his own ultimate goal.

Bach's study of human nature extended far beyond the hospital wards. He found himself categorising people he met socially too, and one evening during a dinner party he realised that all humanity seemed to divide itself up into particular groups of individuals – those who were fearful, those who were doubtful, those who were uncertain, or too concerned, those who were lonely, and those who seemed disinterested or indifferent.

He carried on these observations back in his consulting rooms, and soon began to notice that patients in the same character group responded best to the same type of homoeopathic vaccine (or nosode). There were seven nosodes, and at this stage he had worked out seven character groups: the relationship between them became so obvious that Bach began to base his selection of nosode entirely on the charac-ter and temperament of his patients, and abandoned the clinical exam-ination of bowel flora. This led to even better results, and it was the improved health of chronically sick people that confirmed to him that personality and not disease was the most accurate basis for diagnosis.

Dr Bach then began searching for a harmless, positive, plant-based substitute for the bacterial starting materials he had thus far been work-ing with. He experimented with a selection of flora and began to match the nosodes to specific plants, but he soon understood that he was on the brink of a whole new way of thinking. He realised that what he really wanted to find were plants which would actually heal negative emotional states, and have a direct effect on the personality. He could then offer his patients a treatment not just for certain chronic diseases but instead treat the real root causes of his patients' problems. The task before him was to find a means of preventing ill health by treating mental disharmony at its earliest stage, before it had a chance to manifest itself as physical suffering. Absolutely convinced that this was the path to take, he immediately packed his bags and left his work and London behind him.

This was in 1930. During the course of the six years that followed he discovered and finalised a complete system of medicine specifically intended to relieve emotional suffering and restore harmony and happiness to the personality. This system would free the body from the influence of negative thought, stress, depression, anger etc., so that its own natural healing processes had a proper chance to work.

The complete system Dr Bach discovered is made up of 38 individual remedies. Thirty-seven are prepared from the flowers of plants or trees; one is made from the water of a natural spring. Each remedy addresses a specific state of mind, mood or personality trait: for example, Scleranthus for indecision, Pine for guilt, Clematis for the daydreamer. Remedies can be mixed together in order to address the subtle variations in mood and outlook that exist in every individual, so that in spite of there only being 38 remedies, the system as a whole is capable of covering the needs of every living thing in this world.

The 38 remedies were divided by Dr Bach under seven general headings, each describing a particular emotional category. The seven groups are:
1. Fear
2. Uncertainty
3. Insufficient interest in present circumstances
4. Loneliness
5. Oversensitivity to influences and ideas
6. Despondency or despair
7. Overcare for the welfare of others.

The group headings were derived from Dr Bach's early work with vaccines and nosodes, and although he chose to retain the seven headings, they lost much of their significance when he finalised his work and gave equal importance to the 38 individual emotional states within those groups.

Each one of the individual remedies falls under one of the seven headings. For example, the Fear category consists of five remedies: Rock Rose (for terror), Mimulus (for nervousness about known things),

Cherry Plum (for fear of losing control), Aspen (for vague, causeless apprehension), and Red Chestnut (for over-anxiousness about the well-being of someone else).

The system is designed to be easy to use. When you begin to think about helping yourself or your animal, you first need to identify which of the 38 remedies are appropriate. If you find it hard to pinpoint the precise difficulty, try to identify in general terms with the problem as a whole. The group heading may be of assistance in this respect, and once you have determined which group category best suits your needs, let it act as a doorway to the more detailed exploration of the individual remedies. However, do not worry if you are unable to relate to the group – the individual remedy choice is far more important and precise.

As you read the remedy indications (see page 17–39) you will notice that some remedies describe personality traits – the characteristics which make individual people and animals who they are. Examples are Agrimony (for people who put a brave face on their troubles) and Rock Water (for people who strive for self-perfection and hope others might learn by following their example). Other remedies only describe moods or emotions which, whilst commonly experienced by us all, do not relate specifically to our character or personality. Examples include Star of Bethlehem (for shock and a sense of loss) and Mustard (for despondency with no known cause). In any case, all of the remedies address states of mind which every one of us might encounter from time to time as we go through life, but when we are selecting the remedies, we need to isolate the one or the few which are immediately relevant. Therefore we need to identify the most prevalent state(s) of mind, the mood which describes the thing or things that bother us the most.

If the troubling emotion is a mood of the moment or a passing state of mind, then the remedies we select will usually enable us to overcome the negativity and regain a positive outlook quite quickly. But if the problem is one of greater substance, one which has become a deep-seated issue, and has grown with time, then we need to ensure that we select not only those remedies which address the moods which are uppermost in our minds, but also the remedy for our basic personality, that is, our **type remedy**.

For example, if you are someone who enjoys privacy, keeping yourself to yourself, preferring a quiet life, then you are likely to be a Water Violet type. If you are someone who hates to be in a subservient position, instinctively takes charge of situations, leads the way and generally assumes a dominant role, then you are probably a Vine type. The remedy which describes you is your type remedy, and more often than not it will be included as part of your treatment because it is the remedy to help you to regain your personal equilibrium and find your true self again.

When selecting remedies for an animal it is also important, although not always as easy, to identify the correct type remedy. If you know the animal well you are more likely to appreciate its personal little ways, its general demeanour and temperament. You will know whether it is timid and uncertain or boisterous and confident. You will know whether it is a leader or a follower, proud and aloof or possessive and clingy. It is the animal's nature, summed up in these terms, which will guide you in respect of the correct choice of type remedy or remedies, just as these factors would guide you in the choice of your own remedies.

The humanity of animals

Are animals, then, exactly the same as people?

Some think they are, and this belief leads to the assumption that animals and people are able to understand each other's motives, beliefs and behaviour without any need for interpretation. So if we see a horse biting and kicking we should automatically reach for Vine, Holly or Cherry Plum. When human beings bite and kick, they are bullying, or full of hate, or having a tantrum, so the conclusion is that the same must apply to all animals.

Unfortunately things are not that simple. (If they were, cats would know instinctively why we don't want them to climb up the expensive new curtains.) However close we are to animals, and however close animals are to each other, each species has millions of years of differential evolution behind it. The average, normal behaviour of a human being, a wolf and a chicken differ in many basic and subtle ways. What is reasonable for one species, given its special needs and its special evolutionary direction, may seem *un*reasonable to another – and motives are easily misunderstood.

Take a classic example of 'problematic' animal behaviour. A lady owns a dozen cats who all live together reasonably happily. Then she introduces a new cat, a male tom, rescued from the street. Immediately all hell breaks loose. The new cat and the others do not get on, and it seems there is a great deal of spite and viciousness from all of them.

From the owner's point of view there is no need for all of this, and the cats are behaving unreasonably. But seen from the cat's point of view this aggressive behaviour is entirely reasonable, since the cats need to establish for their own peace of mind which is the dominant animal. Once this has been achieved things may settle down (although it could be that there are simply too many cats for the space available, in which case they won't settle down until there is more room or fewer cats).

Cats also provide another example of how anthropomorphism – the idea that the thoughts and actions of an animal can be translated directly into human terms – can lead us astray. Cats, especially toms, occasionally open their mouths, wrinkle their noses and curl their lips in disgust – or at least, that's sometimes how cat owners describe their behaviour. In fact they are gathering smells into a special organ called the vomeronasal organ, and what they are doing is called flehming. It's hard to know exactly what cats experience when they do this because humans don't have a working vomeronasal organ, but the fact that toms flehm most when they are near females in season suggests that disgust isn't an appropriate description.

Similarly, a dog's nose is far more sensitive than ours. Dogs 'see' into a complex world of odour that we cannot even begin to describe in words. Bats use echo location – a sense we don't seem to possess at all – so what exactly is it like to be a bat? We cannot say.

We need to be aware then of the fundamental differences between us and other animals and between different species of animals if we are to be successful when selecting remedies for them. One way to do this is to give a little thought to the basic personality of the particular species we are dealing with. For example, horses are herd animals, so they like to be with other horses. A horse by itself in a field will probably feel isolated and scared. They are also prey animals, so a fear reaction to a strange human is not unreasonable. They prefer to live in open spaces and don't like to be shut in, for their response to fear is to run away. Knowing this, the response of a race horse forced into a starting stall suddenly becomes entirely understandable. It isn't stubbornness or pig-headedness that makes the animal unwilling to enter the stall, but fear.

The same factors – social behaviour (or lack of it), prey or predator, and natural habitat – can be analysed for any species so as to provide a general description of the average mindset of that kind of animal. For example, knowing that rabbits are more likely to feel fear than pure aggression helps to define rabbit behaviour in general. Individual animals may still need Vine for overdominant behaviour, particularly when interacting within their own groups, but the species-specific description should make inappropriate uses of such remedies less likely.

This method will not resolve the problem of understanding an animal's mind, but at least it points a way forward. And while we need to keep in mind the differences between species we also need to guard against going too far the other way, and making difference an excuse for lack of empathy. For all the differences between living things, there are also basic similarities. We share organs – heart, liver, brain, eyes – and we share the basic structure of life, death and reproduction as well.

We also share emotions, something which is poignantly captured in a distressing true story – told by Bruce Fogle in his book *The Dog's Mind* – of what happened when a cow elephant died in a safari park. A pathologist decided to do a full post-mortem on the large dead animal, and because of the difficulty involved in trying to move it he decided to do the examination on the spot where it had died.

As the work got underway the pathologist needed to move the large, dismembered pieces around the shed. A bull elephant, the dead cow's mate, was brought in to help shift them. First it was made to pick up and move one of the legs, which it did, although it seemed agitated. Then it had to move the cow's head – again, it did as it was told, but beat its trunk in the air and trumpeted once it had done so. After this the door was opened and the elephant was allowed to leave. It ran outside and as far away as possible from the shed, pressed its head onto the ground and trumpeted for a long time. It did not move again until its trainer came up and spoke to it.

Can you select remedies for this animal? We think you can: Star of Bethlehem, certainly, for the shock and grief of what happened; and Rock Rose for the terror and extreme fright. Both are in Rescue Remedy, of course. Elephants care for their mates: why should it be surprising that all the problems associated with human grief can also arise in elephants? So Sweet Chestnut could be added for the great anguish felt.

The fact is that the brains of all mammals – including our own and an elephant's – are so similar that it is simpler to hypothesise that animals **do** have emotions than it is to deny their existence. This means that Occam's razor, a respected scientific principle that prefers the simpler of two theories, supports the unscientific belief that we can and should understand this elephant's pain.

Nowadays more and more animal behaviourists in the West have come to reject narrow behaviourism and give credence to the more subjective, anthropomorphic approach that has long been the tradition in the East. And when you think about it, this is only right and proper. After all, in our hearts we know that animals think and feel: we can measure the REM rates of dreaming dogs and predict the erratic behaviour of cats when their owners take them off to a new house where they feel unsettled. Science has yet to find a satisfactory way of measuring human emotion, and no doubt it will take even longer to measure animal emotions – but that is no reason not to use the empathetic gifts we all have to help animals as well as humans.

Of course, we are especially lucky because we have extra proof of the usefulness of anthropomorphism and subjectivity in understanding animal emotions: the fact that we can select Bach Flower Remedies for them and see them feel better. Every time a grieving dog is successfully given Star of Bethlehem or an unsettled cat benefits from Walnut then we know that our subjectivity has led us aright.

Do animals have souls?

This is where another interesting question about animals surfaces. Dr Bach describes the remedies and writes about their actions and benefits as they relate to human beings. His patients were people not animals, and it was the health and well-being of the people he saw during his working life who were the focus of his concerns. In his writings he was quite specific about how the remedies could help people but for many the idea that these remedies can work in the same way for animals is unsettling, not to say controversial.

This may come as a surprise to those who consider giving remedies to animals to be as natural as taking remedies themselves, but giving Bach Flower Remedies to animals is different from, say, giving a vitamin supplement or using an accepted therapy like acupuncture, which has been used on animals in China for thousands of years. This is because using the remedies could be seen as being the same as saying that animals not only have individual personalities, but have souls as well.

Why is this?

Dr Bach believed that there are different facets of our existence on earth. On the one hand there is our earth-bound personality, which is the side of our selves that we see and act with every day. On the other there is our higher self, which is our spiritual, eternal side. The higher self is not incarnated directly on earth, but acts through the personality instead.

The personality has a limited autonomy of its own. It can choose to live a correct and profitable life in accordance with the evolutionary needs of the higher self; or it can go astray and act in ways that damage those needs. It can also act with cruelty, or selfishness or hatred, all of which are actions that work against the divine principle of the unity of all things.

Dr Bach saw illness as one of the methods that the higher self uses to correct the defects of the personality. As long as the personality is acting in accordance with the principle of unity, and in accordance with the aims of the higher self, then there can be no illness. But when the personality goes wrong, that is the trigger for ill health to appear.

The role of the remedies in this scheme is to help the personality to see where it is going wrong. So if hatred is the problem causing the personality to act against unity, then Holly can be used. This remedy is allied to the natural quality or emotion of love, so taking the remedy strengthens the virtue within us and washes out the fault. The personality is once more in harmony with unity and the illness no longer has a role to play.

Similarly, if the personality is overfearful and overprotective of others, to the extent that the anxiety felt is hampering not only the evolutionary needs of the higher self but also the needs of the people being worried over, then the remedy Red Chestnut can be used to reinforce the calming, comforting side of us which can help others without provoking anxiety.

Because the higher self is our immortal part it is, in effect, the same as the soul, so the action of the remedies can be described as putting the personality back in tune with the soul. Consequently if the remedies are given to animals, the imputation is that animals have souls and personalities just like people.

Pet owners would all agree that animals do have personalities, and we have seen that in the past behaviourists would not. But nowadays this is not the case. A few years ago, for example, a piece appeared in the academic journal *Animal Behaviour* in which three scientists who were studying cat behaviour wrote: 'We felt that each animal in our laboratory colony had a distinct personality in the sense that the sum total of its behaviour gave it an identifiable style.' In other words, they were saying that the cats had their own personalities. This is of course what every cat owner believes to be the case.

One of the most respected animal behaviourists of modern times was Konrad Lorenz. This is what he wrote in his book *On Agression*: 'If it is argued that animals are not persons, I must reply by saying that personality begins where, of two individuals, each one plays in the life of the other a part that cannot easily be played by any other member of the species. In other words, personality begins where personal bonds are formed for the first time.' In the same book, Lorenz talks quite openly – and without inverted commas – of geese falling in love with each other, of close friends who have quarrelled being too embarrassed to look at each other, and of manifestations of jealousy. 'All the objectively observable characteristics of the goose's behaviour on losing its mate are roughly identical with those accompanying human grief' he writes. 'We are convinced that animals do have emotions.' (Remember the elephant?)

So much for personality – what now about the existence of animal souls? It is a question that has been debated for centuries in religious circles, and not one to be settled here – but again there is no shortage of supporters of the view that animals do have souls. From the past we could mention Hippocrates ('The soul is the same in all living creatures, although the body of each is different'), and Pythagorus ('Animals share with us the privilege of having a soul'); and more recently there are many thousands of veterinary surgeons who have reached the same conclusion. To mention just one, Dr Patrick Glidden, an American vet, is quoted in the December 1997 issue of *Life* magazine as saying: 'I believe that after euthanasia an animal's soul leaves his or her body and goes to the Creator. Animals are such innocents. Why wouldn't God want to surround Himself with their goodness – the goodness of creations that didn't reject Him, as we did?'

Even if you don't accept these views, the lack of a theoretical construct should not be enough to stop you using the remedies to treat animals. In fact, many of the most commonly used 'orthodox' medicines work in ways that we do not understand. Nobody knows, for example, how aspirin works, and the pharmacological action of some antibiotics is equally mysterious. No one is seriously saying that we should stop using aspirin because we don't know how it works: and the same argument must apply to complementary medicines. All the more so, as the Bach Flower Remedies, unlike aspirin, are all non-toxic, gentle and safe.

So one doesn't necessarily have to agree with Dr Bach's view of the soul and personality, nor does one need to believe that animals have souls, in order to use the remedies. The plain fact is that whether or not the person using them believes in them, the remedies work. And whether animals have souls or not, the remedies work on animals. As Dr Bach himself said 'no science, no knowledge is necessary ... and they who will obtain the greatest benefit from this God-sent gift will be those who keep it pure as it is; free from science, free from theories, for everything in Nature is simple.' The way is clear to start using the remedies. Let's learn how to do this.

CHAPTER 2:

Using The Remedies

The role for the remedies

For many years, and not that long ago, Western medicine treated the physical body alone. In effect this meant dealing with physical symptoms. Most people accepted this concept of medicine as self-evident common sense. The metaphor used to explain the way bodies worked was a mechanical one. Something was broken; it had to be fixed. Thinking about how an animal – porcine or bovine, feline or human – felt on an emotional level was at best sentimental and at worst downright counterproductive, in that it got in the way of the impersonal judgement expected of the professional in charge of the case.

It hadn't always been this way. In ancient times learned men such as Paracelsus and Hippocrates attributed value to the personal approach, looking beyond the physical to the whole being on a mental, emotional and spiritual level. This led to rules such as Paracelsus' dictum that the wise physician should treat five rather than fifteen patients in a day, and to the valuing of living things generally as mental and spiritual beings.

In our own times this view of the world has given rise to complementary medicine. The word often used to describe this approach is **holistic**: the idea that the whole person is implicated in wellness or illness, not just the body, and that because of this it is important to treat the whole being.

The concept of holism has spread far beyond the consulting rooms of individual complementary practitioners. The vast majority of orthodox doctors would now acknowledge that a really successful treatment will include therapies and approaches aimed at helping the person to be happier and more fulfilled. Health today means more than the ability to function simply on a physical level.

Even within the holistic world of complementary medicine, however, Dr Bach's system of medicine is unique. It is the only one that is aimed solely at emotions and mental states, and the only one that takes no account whatsoever of any physical complaints that the sufferer has.

Because of this approach the system of 38 remedies is uniquely equipped to deal with emotional unhappiness. Cats having to get used to new homes, dogs pining for their former owners, horses terrified of humans after being mistreated, all are obvious candidates for remedies that will deal with these emotional imbalances, and so restore confidence to the first, joy to the second, and courage to the third.

This is not to say that the remedies cannot also be useful when there is a physical problem. An unstressed, happy and balanced animal is always going to be healthier, and will recover better from illness, than an animal that is stressed, unhappy and out of balance. Whether the problem is ringworm or a broken leg or distemper, then, animals can be given remedies alongside whatever other treatment they are receiving, remedies that will not themselves kill the worms, set the leg or cure the distemper, but will help animals to feel better in themselves, freeing their bodies to find their own natural state of health.

Because the remedies can be used alongside other forms of treatment they are really complementary rather than alternative medicines. This means that you can use whatever orthodox or alternative treatment is appropriate for any physical problems the animal is suffering from, while at the same time treating the animal's personality and emotional imbalances with the remedies. This makes the remedies very flexible to use and means that the best treatment remains available for specific physical disorders.

Sometimes people take this a step further and try to use the remedies directly for specific illnesses. When treating human beings they will give Rock Water (for rigidity of mind) to all those suffering from arthritis and other forms of physical rigidity, or they will select White Chestnut for all cases of insomnia on the assumption that insomnia is always and only due to worrying mental arguments. This is a mistake, of course, and shows a lack of understanding of the basics of this system of healing. It really is best to leave the diagnosis and treatment of physical conditions to the people qualified to carry them out – in the case of animals, the vet.

The 38 remedies

In order to use the remedies to their fullest potential you will need to familiarise yourself as much as possible with their indications. Once you know them well you will find that you are drawn to those which you or your animals need, almost without hesitation. Your motivation will be greater when you know you do not have to spend time reading the indications of all 38 in order to select the ones you need. You will save yourself time, the system will be more useable, and you will turn to it more regularly once you know the remedies well.

We have set out below the indications for each of the 38 remedies, giving first the general (human) factors, followed by a description of how the remedy relates specifically to animals. This will help you to appreciate the qualities of each remedy. The remedies have been set out in alphabetical order as this makes them easier to find, so that you can refer to and re-read remedy descriptions as necessary – first during the course of your study of this book, and again later on when you start to use the remedies for real.

AGRIMONY
For those who hide their suffering behind a mask of cheerfulness.
Human beings of this nature tend to be gregarious, happy, fun-loving people. They dislike making a fuss and so conceal their anxiety, depression, pain, grief or bad temper behind their usual bonny exterior and cheerful personality. No one would know that they were suffering such inner torture, they hide it so well.

Animals of the Agrimony disposition will also be naturally happy-go-lucky. They will enjoy your laughter at their antics, and will be sensitive to arguments or any bad feeling in the household. If you are distressed, your Agrimony companion will be distressed too. But instead of looking dejected or crying for attention he is likely to play the court jester, making all sorts of attempts to divert your attention from the object of your upset and, despite his own suffering, try to make you happy again.

ASPEN
Vague or unaccountable fears and apprehension. Fear of the unknown.
Human beings suffering this state of mind will tell you that they feel afraid, as though something is about to happen, but they cannot identify what it is that makes them feel this way. They are on tenterhooks

and are jumpy as though they are living on a knife-edge, full of fearful anticipation. They are anxious but do not know why.

Animals in the Aspen state may suddenly start to whine, pant or appear agitated for no apparent reason. The fear may begin in their sleep as night terrors or they may wake up in this state. Equally it may happen at any time of the day, and there may be a ghostly, apprehensive look in the animal's eyes. But there will be no obvious trigger – nothing to which you can say: 'he gets like this whenever so-and-so happens' or 'this is how he reacts to next door's cat ever since she scratched him.' If your animal has bouts of fear for no specific reason, Aspen is likely to be the remedy he needs.

BEECH
Criticism of and intolerance towards other people, events and situations. Lack of understanding.

Beech people think of themselves as perfectionists. They believe that their way is the only sensible one and have no leniency towards other people who do things differently. Beech people are irritated by the idiosyncrasies of others. They consider other people to be a nuisance or stupid, and fail to appreciate that everyone has an equal right to live and learn from personal beliefs, mistakes and experiences.

In order to determine when an animal might need Beech, we need to look for evidence of intolerance towards people and other animals, or towards events and situations. In the first instance, there may be an obvious dislike of a particular person or particular animal, perhaps with evidence of other remedy traits too such as jealousy (Holly) or a desire to dominate (Vine). In the second, there may be intolerance of getting into the car, for example, or going to certain houses or wearing a lead.

CENTAURY
Kind-hearted and eager to please, but weak-willed and unable to say no or set limits.

People of this nature find it hard to stand up for themselves. They are easily dominated, and because it is in their nature to want to be of help this willingness can easily be exploited. They then find themselves in situations that they do not enjoy, or doing something they do not want to do simply because they do not have the strength to say no.

Animals of a Centaury nature, like their human counterparts, are gentle, caring souls. They are obedient, will always do as they are told and are very rarely naughty. They will fetch, carry, and sit for hours.

Dogs of this nature obey everyone and so make hopeless guards. Placid horses who are never any trouble may be Centaury horses. Cats who get picked on by a pack leader along the road and come home injured or bedraggled but uncomplaining may also be Centauries. And kittens or puppies of this nature are the ones who don't assert themselves and may fail to thrive because they get pushed out of the way at feed times.

CERATO

Doubtful distrust of one's own judgement or interpretation.

People of the Cerato type do not really trust themselves, or more exactly they do not trust their own minds. They ask others what to do because they have no faith in their own instincts. This self-doubt may occur in a variety of circumstances, from what to wear to how to handle a situation. Underneath it all these people know what they want but they question their judgement and find themselves seeking confirmation from friends before making their decision and taking the final step.

Animals of the Cerato disposition, like children of this nature, may look at you before acting in order to see what you want them to do. Rather than act of their own accord they will wait for your confirmation that it's OK to go ahead.

CHERRY PLUM

Fear of insanity; loss of mental control.

Although extreme, the Cherry Plum state is one most people will have experienced to some extent – the feeling that you are going crazy. It may be the result of anything from the children getting under your feet to complete paranoia. Basically, it is an overwhelming sense of losing your grip on a situation so that you become frightened that you will snap and do something irrational or inappropriate, perhaps with disastrous consequences.

Animals, like people, may suffer from an isolated Cherry Plum state, but it is more likely that it will be linked to or be a by-product of something else. For example, a cat who cleans obsessively to the point of self-mutilation would need Crab Apple for the overriding desire for cleanliness and the obsessive behaviour, and Cherry Plum because of the loss of control associated with self-injury. Similarly, any animal suffering with an irritating condition or infection may lose its self-control until the irritation is eased, and violently scratch itself in a desperate attempt to find relief.

CHESTNUT BUD

Inability to learn from past mistakes.

This remedy is for those who take a long time to learn from experience. They repeat the same error and stumble into the same pitfalls again and again, often without acknowledging the fact that they have done it all before. They might make errors of judgement such as moving house because living near a railway line is too noisy, only to move into another house just as close to another railway line. They may keep failing an exam on the same point, or become ill from repeatedly eating food they know disagrees with them. On a deeper level, they may not progress in life because they are unable to recognise, and thus correct, a fundamental fault in their own personality. Whatever the problem, it is the repetition of mistakes that Chestnut Bud addresses, enabling the individual to learn from experience and so move on in life.

Animals, too, may have difficulty learning and so may repeat the same unsuccessful behaviour patterns or may fail to grasp a new skill. An animal that is reprimanded for unsociable behaviour such as chewing the cushions, yet continues to chew cushions no matter how many times he is told not to, may be a candidate for Chestnut Bud. Similarly, an animal who is rewarded for using the litter tray and yet nine times out of ten fails to use it despite the rewards when he does, may also benefit from this remedy. Another example may be when a horse continues to knock down the same fence in the arena, even though it is well within its capabilities. Or the cat who teases another cat and is viciously attacked in return, but continues the same behaviour, despite similar and repeated retaliation, all the time apparently unaware of the relationship between his action and the other cat's response.

Chestnut Bud may need to be combined with other remedies in some instances, but it is the key remedy whenever repetition prevents progress.

CHICORY

Possessiveness, selfishness.

The positive side of the Chicory nature is one of great love and warmth. The negative aspect is shown when the Chicory person begins to manipulate, feign affection and use emotional blackmail to get his or her own way.

The key to Chicory people is that they feel that they deserve appreciation in return for the concern they show others – especially members of their own family – and always expect to be the centre of attention.

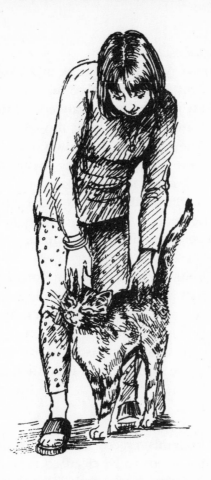

They feel hurt and are easily offended if their advice is not taken or if they feel that they are not being treated with enough respect. They can be full of self-pity if they do not feel loved or appreciated. In this latter respect, Chicory may combine well with Willow, which is the remedy specifically for self-pity, resentment and bitterness.

Chicory animals are also possessive in nature, and in their positive state are very loving companions. You can recognise a Chicory animal because it will be the one who sits near you, demanding your attention and to be petted, especially if anyone else should enter the room. A cat who rubs against your legs constantly and follows you everywhere may well be a Chicory cat. Chicory is the remedy for caring too much, so Chicory animals are territorial creatures and will be highly protective of their family and home. They will enjoy preparing their nest and can be especially possessive when it comes to protecting their young or their possessions.

CLEMATIS

Daydreaming, mental escapism.

People of the Clematis type appear to be in a world of their own. In conversation you might suddenly realise they are not listening to what you have to say – their minds have wandered and become absorbed by some fantasy adventure or pleasant thoughts of some wished-for future happening. They tend to be drowsy individuals who can fall asleep almost anywhere and at any time. They may find it difficult to concentrate, perhaps reading the same page of a book again and again because their minds drift, so that they awake to find themselves thinking of something else entirely. This is also the remedy indicated for the numb, bemused state of mind which precipitates or follows a fainting attack.

In animals the same indications apply. You may notice that your companion is unusually (or maybe usually) distant. For example, there may be a vacant look in the eyes, which seem to be staring at nothing. Animals who seem to sleep all the time or have trouble paying attention or those who seem, for whatever reason, to live more in a dream than in the present – all these might benefit from Clematis.

CRAB APPLE

The cleansing remedy.

Those who benefit from this remedy feel there is something unpleasant about themselves that needs to be cleansed from their system. It may be a sense of contamination, for example if they have come into contact with infection or poison, or they may feel disgusted with themselves for having overeaten. In the Crab Apple state, these feelings are much greater than the mild distaste that most people would experience in similar circumstances, and can escalate to obsession or compulsion. When ill, Crab Apple people feel diseased and contaminated by whatever is wrong with them. Any disfigurement, blemish or symptom is exaggerated in their minds, and because they have a general tendency to be overconcerned with detail and trivialities they dwell on minor symptoms to the exclusion of everything else.

Another characteristic of Crab Apple people is that they dislike the way they look and so think of themselves as ugly. They may be revolted by their own bodies and those of others – bodily functions offend Crab Apple people greatly. They cannot bear to be dirty or to live in a dirty environment and so tend to be overly house-proud, obsessively tidying and cleaning.

This overdesire for cleanliness is evident in animals who display excessive grooming habits. Cats and dogs who constantly lick themselves or nibble obsessively at their fur could benefit from Crab Apple. Others that seem to have a distaste for eating or mating or defecating might benefit as well.

ELM
Overwhelmed with responsibility.
People of the Elm type are often found in positions of responsibility. They are capable people, who do not lack confidence and are perfectly able and willing to deal with all sorts of situations. However, if they take on additional duties or are burdened with extra responsibility, such as might happen following promotion, they can suddenly become overwhelmed by the thought of what is expected of them. This is when they begin to lose their confidence, feel despondent and doubt their ability to cope; and this is when Elm is needed to restore confidence and positive thought and remind them of their capabilities.

Animals with Elm indications will be those who feel burdened by a sense of responsibility. This may include dogs, cats and horses who take part in shows and who may normally be quite confident creatures, but suddenly panic when about to enter the arena, and shy away and display other signs of distress. Rescue Remedy would be helpful for stage fright, but Elm should be an additional consideration, especially if this behaviour occurs in normally reliable and steady animals.

Elm would also be useful for a mother who abandons her litter because she cannot face or cope with the expectations of her young. Guide dogs and hearing dogs may also need Elm from time to time. They are chosen for their capable, calm and dependable temperament, but there may be occasions, perhaps noticeable during training sessions, when they appear to lose their confidence and calm and when the responsibility which is placed upon them becomes a burden.

GENTIAN
Despondency, discouragement.
Whenever a setback has made someone feel unhappy, doubtful, downhearted or depressed, Gentian is the remedy to restore optimism. It brings encouragement and positive thought, thus preventing a sense of hopelessness from developing.

Animals who need Gentian will also have encountered a setback – perhaps they have lost an event in the gymkhana, or have been separated from their owner or a companion, or have been told they will not be going for their usual walk today. Whenever there is discouragement or when a mildly depressed feeling occurs for a particular reason, then Gentian is the remedy to choose.

GORSE
Hopelessness, pessimism.

The Gorse despondency is deeper than that of Gentian. Put simply, in the Gentian state of mind people feel on the verge of giving up; in the Gorse state they *have* given up. There may still be an exit route, but people in the Gorse state do not believe one exists. Quite often they refuse to look for a solution, claiming that nothing can be done for them, and because they feel so negative, it is difficult, if not impossible, to persuade them otherwise.

Animals cannot tell you that they feel hopeless, but you may recognise the fact from their facial expressions and body language. A dog in the Gorse state will probably hold its tail between its legs and its head down, and may appear more introverted than usual. It will *look* heavy-hearted.

This frame of mind might be most noticeable when the animal is ill. Some animals may look as though they have given up hope and are ready to die, but by giving Gorse quite often the spirits are lifted, optimism returns, and consequently there is a greater chance of recovery from the illness.

HEATHER
Self-absorption.

The Heather type of person is one who needs company and someone to talk to. However, the conversation is one-sided because people who would benefit from the Heather remedy do not listen to what other people have to say, nor are they particularly interested. They are preoccupied with their own problems, families and lives. On the positive side, Heather people are very sociable and never stuck for something to say, but encountering a negative Heather type is an exhausting and suffocating experience. They talk at you and not to you.

If the Heather person is not interested in what you have to say, however, there is still one thing that he does want from you. Heather people cannot handle loneliness and must have an audience, so they want to keep you with them at all costs. And again your needs do not count. Sometimes you might have plenty of time to give and no other pressing engagements, but the Heather person is just as likely to corner you in a busy supermarket, at the front door, in the street, over the garden fence, at the doctor's surgery, or at any other moment when you have something else you have to attend to. It simply wouldn't occur to the Heather person that you might have something better to do. And this is why people tend to avoid Heather folk. Their tragedy is that by their behaviour they bring about the very thing they are desperate to avoid: loneliness.

Heather animals are also overconcerned with companionship. They may constantly bark or whimper or grunt to ensure that you aware of their presence; they may make noises when you have a visitor, or may get overexcited when someone calls at the house, presenting the caller with toys etc., or by using some other method to get attention. When a Heather animal is left alone it will whine incessantly and watch and wait, hour upon hour, for your return. Sometimes it can be difficult to distinguish between the need to use Chicory or Heather because there is an element of selfishness in both remedy types, but with Heather there is no pride or cunning as would be the case with the Chicory type. Heather motivation is innocent and clear, driven only by the desire for company. Furthermore the source of attention is less important for Heather animals: they will take attention from any casual visitor and even hang around people who obviously do not want them there; Chicory animals will prefer the people they are close to, and will stalk off full of resentment and wounded pride if they are snubbed.

HOLLY
Jealousy, envy, hatred, suspicion.
Holly is the remedy for vexations – those emotions which erode the soul, those which fill one's thoughts with a desire for revenge. Holly emotions are devoid of love, and are based around strong negative feelings directed at others.

Holly relates to animals in the same way as it relates to humans, although animals may show their emotions more clearly than humans. Spitefulness, for example, may amount to the odd caustic remark or muttered aside in human beings, but in animals it is likely to be more obvious – growling, hissing, barking, snapping and unprovoked attacks. Jealousy may be apparent, perhaps due to the arrival of a new animal or a new baby into the household, indeed anyone who apparently threatens existing relationships; and in such cases the displaced animal may try to reassert itself by showing hostility to the intruder. Vine could be considered for this situation, either instead of or along with Holly.

There is an important fact to bear in mind when considering the use of this remedy, which is that Holly is probably the most overused remedy there is when it comes to helping animals. As we will see later on in this book, aggression in most animals, certainly when directed at humans, is far more likely to be based on fear than on hatred.

HONEYSUCKLE
Preoccupation with memories of the past.
This is the remedy for those who are unable to give their full attention to the present, but instead dwell on happy memories and the good times they once had. It is because they believe that life will never be as good again that they allow the past to dominate their thoughts.

Animals would need Honeysuckle for the same reasons – when they long for what has gone. The remedy might be considered if the animal shows signs of distress – becoming introverted, losing its appetite etc. – when it has been parted from someone or somewhere it knows and trusts.

HORNBEAM
Lethargy, unaccountable mental weariness.
The Hornbeam state is often described as 'the Monday morning feeling'. It is the cloud of weary lassitude which makes us feel as though we have no strength to face the day or task ahead, and leads us to procrastinate or give up the job altogether. The Hornbeam remedy helps to remove that languor thus enabling us to look upon life's challenges more eagerly, more willingly and with a greater sense of purpose.

Animals can also suffer this Hornbeam state of mind. An animal who seems to be lazy, shying away from anything which is demanding or requiring activity, for example a dog lacking enthusiasm to go for a walk, may be in the Hornbeam state (although there are other remedies such as Wild Rose which should also be considered). The way to recognise Hornbeam is through the weariness.

Signs of fatigue alone may lead you to think of Olive in the first instance, but the Olive tiredness always has a reason, essentially over-work. With Hornbeam, there is no actual reason – it is tiredness at the *thought* of doing something rather than feeling tired due to the effort of actually having done it.

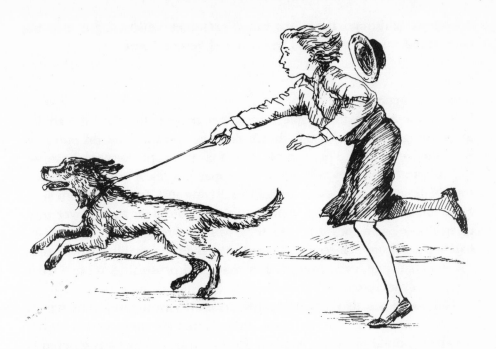

IMPATIENS

Impatience, quick-mindedness, irritability.

Impatiens people are generally of high intellectual ability, and think clearly and directly about whatever they set their minds to. They prefer to be left to work alone and at their own pace. That way they do not feel hampered or restrained by the presence of other people. They like the freedom to move ahead and get on with the job in hand, so they find interruptions irritating. Similarly their quick minds have little room for idle chat – they will discuss what needs to be discussed, but will then want to close the conversation quickly and get on without delay.

At their most positive, Impatiens people are intelligent, clear-minded, open and to-the-point, with a quick-witted sense of humour. Their negative disposition is one of tension, agitation, impatience and irritation at the methodical slowness, indecision, apathy and triviality of other people. In their hurry they may jump to conclusions or miss vital information, and their desire to do things quickly can mean that they put themselves under unnecessary pressure.

In animals, the Impatiens indications would be largely behavioural – cats that are always rushing about, dogs that cannot wait to be taken out for a walk and always run on ahead, and generally animals that seem to have endless energy. Horses who are difficult to control before a race or a show may be impatient for the event to begin and so may need

Impatiens (although there are other remedies which might also be considered, such as Mimulus, Vervain and Rescue Remedy).

LARCH

Lack of self-confidence.

Larch is the remedy for people who do not believe they have the ability to do things. Because of this they hold back and miss out on much of what life has to offer. For example, they may not apply for a job because they do not think they will get it. They may not learn to drive because they believe they are bound to fail the driving test. In a classroom situation children of the Larch type would not volunteer the answer to a question because they are sure they will be wrong and look foolish. Larch people are self-conscious and retreat from anything which presents a challenge, even though they may (and probably do) have what it takes to succeed.

Larch animals also lack self-confidence and avoid situations where they might have to perform. Larch animals that are presented at shows may be subdued prior to the event, for example, or shy away when it is their turn, or walk into the arena head down and tail between the legs. Refusing relatively simple jumps may be a horse's way of dealing with lack of self-esteem – better to refuse to jump than to jump badly.

Another situation where the remedy might be helpful is when a cat is obliged to integrate into an existing feline social structure, and may feel daunted and unsure of itself because of this. And for the same reason animals that have been rescued from bad homes might also need this remedy to help them regain their confidence.

MIMULUS

Shyness, timidity, everyday fears of known things.

Fear of crowds, fear of people and of being in the public eye are all characteristics of the Mimulus type, who tends to be shy and timid. As a mood remedy, Mimulus is for anyone who suffers from a fear that can be identified clearly – fear of pain, poverty, spiders, of being killed in an accident, of being burgled etc.

Fear of failure is a Larch indication (see above) as it suggests a lack of confidence in one's ability to succeed; but Mimulus fear of the consequences may be more specific such as fear of what people might say, or fear of having to make the winner's speech. As this suggests, it is not always easy to draw a clear line between Larch and Mimulus, and they are often given together. The normal way to tell them apart is this: if there is a lack of confidence but no actual anxiety, give Larch alone; if there is a fear of something specific but away from this the person is confident of his or her abilities, then give Mimulus alone.

Animals that need Mimulus as a type remedy are fearful, nervous creatures. They may demonstrate their fear quite openly by shaking or shivering or using other body language when confronted with the thing that frightens them: animals that whimper or hide behind the settee when a stranger enters the house are very likely to be in need of Mimulus.

Animals that are afraid of thunder, fireworks, other animals, or the cracking of wood burning in the grate would all benefit from Mimulus. The remedy should also be considered (as should Centaury and Larch) for animals who find it difficult to assert themselves; but where there is sheer terror, or the fear is not of something specific, other remedies will apply – see the indications for Rock Rose and Aspen.

MUSTARD
Unexplained depression.
The Mustard type of depression is like the descent of a dark cloud that blocks out the light and joy of life. Sufferers cannot explain why they feel this way. Often they have everything to live for and be happy about, yet for some unknown reason they feel tearful, flat and gloomy. Nothing seems to help. There might be a momentary lifting of the mood but the weight of the cloud is too great for it to stay away for long. Typically, the Mustard depression does lift again of its own accord, and just as suddenly as it came, it goes. In some cases it may come and go in cycles, for which see also Scleranthus, but there will never be an everyday explanation for it, such as a lost job or missed opportunity.

Animals in the Mustard state will show signs of depression such as loss of appetite, lethargy, emotionless expression, tail/ears down etc. Certainly it would be right to consider giving Mustard if you do not know why the animal is behaving this way (and also take it to the vet as these symptoms may indicate a physical problem). If the depression has happened before this in itself is highly suggestive of the Mustard state and your choice of remedy can then be made with more certainty.

OAK
Resilience.
Oak people have great strength of character. They are not demanding or forceful, but rather they are reliable, dependable and tend to wrap

others in reassurance and make them feel secure. Oak people keep calm in a crisis and always seem to know what to do for the best. On a personal level they enjoy their independence and dislike being ill or incapacitated as it interferes with their desire to get on with life. Therefore, they will struggle on, despite their pain or discomfort, and may then become exhausted. If forced to rest they feel dissatisfied, irritated and despondent at the restrictions imposed upon them. They are true fighters when it comes to getting well. They do not give in, but maintain a positive outlook – something which is undoubtedly a great help to them during convalescence, so long as they are patient and allows their bodies a chance to heal.

Oak type animals have a similar strength of character and they too show tremendous resilience and resistance when they fall ill. When forced to rest, they try to resist and repeatedly attempt to get up and walk about, no matter how weak they may feel. They will not normally complain, but may show signs of depression or exhaustion. Oak animals, like their human counterparts, are calm and steady rather than excitable. This is what can help tell them apart from Impatiens, Vervain and Vine types, who also have strong characters but demonstrate them in different ways.

OLIVE

Exhaustion due to overwork.

This remedy is for those who have worked hard and as a result feel drained of energy. The tiredness may be mental or physical, recent or long-term, and there may be associated factors such as a personality type predisposed to overwork. But the common denominator and key guiding factor to this remedy is that there is a real reason for the fatigue. It may be due to physical hard toil such as heavy manual labour, or due to studying or doing some other exacting mental work, or it may occur following ill health when the body is both physically and mentally depleted.

In animals, once again the indications are the same. The remedy may be required following ill health, or after an operation, or after the animal has given birth. It may also be helpful for working animals such as sheep dogs and shire horses, or for those who are involved in racing, competitive events or shows, where the demands of taking part and travelling to and fro take their toll. The remedy would also be a help to animals who have suffered and become exhausted through ill management or mistreatment.

PINE
Guilt, self-reproach.
Pine is for people who blame themselves, and who even take the blame for the mistakes of others. They tend to apologise frequently and are hard on themselves in an attempt to correct their perceived misdeeds or negligence. The remedy is indicated whenever guilt is apparent, whether it is due to a recent happening or is concerned with a long-standing and deep-rooted guilt complex.

Animals may also feel guilty at times, but as with Holly, many animals are given Pine inappropriately. If you shout at your puppy for destroying your best shoes, it may look ashamed by averting its eyes, but the actual emotion felt is more likely to be submission and fear. Mimulus is a more helpful choice in these circumstances. An animal that is constantly repremanded may need Pine if it begins to think that everything is its fault, but in general the Pine state is more likely to exist between animals – cat and cat, dog and dog, horse and horse – since there the emotion would not be swamped by our overwhelming dominance.

RED CHESTNUT
Over anxiety for the well-being of others.
Most people will have experienced anxiety, to some extent, for those they care about – perhaps they are worried about a family member who is away from home, or a child going on a school trip for the first time. This is natural parental concern and does not in itself indicate a problem.

The Red Chestnut fear is a similar concern, but exaggerated to the extreme. People in the Red Chestnut state are frantic with worry until they know their loved one is safe. They fret before their partner or child leaves the house and will continue to fret until he or she is back home.

Red Chestnut people are inclined to telephone every day to make sure their loved ones are well and have not come to any harm, and this behaviour can sometimes be confused with the overconcern of Chicory. The difference is that Red Chestnut people are afraid, rather than possessive, and are not concerned at all about themselves – their anxiety is entirely focussed on someone else.

Red Chestnut animals may be difficult to distinguish from those of the Chicory or of the Mimulus type. One way to identify them is to look for something of a cross between the two: nervous, fearful behaviour when you show signs of leaving, combined with an effort to go with you or prevent you from leaving. A mother with her pups or kittens may show intense anxiety if one strays – again, this is indicative of Red Chestnut behaviour.

ROCK ROSE
Terror, panic.

This remedy is for intense fear, so great that it causes the sufferer to feel terrified. There is always a reason for the fear – it may be due to something the person has witnessed, or it may be due to a forthcoming event, or a phobia, or a nightmare, or stem from some terrifying ordeal. Whatever the reason, the fear is specific but has gone beyond the everyday nature of Mimulus. When terror is present, Rock Rose is the remedy to turn to.

When an animal is panic-stricken, physical signs are usually the key to the state of mind. Fur bristles on the back, the stance is one of defence, the expression is stunned or anxious. The whole body may be trembling. These are outward signs of terror, and in certain respects, are no different to the physical symptoms human beings exhibit when they encounter a situation which generates this state of mind. Thunderstorms and fireworks are common causes do a Rock Rose state in animals, but there are other less obvious triggers too, such as visiting the vet, being taken to kennels, or travelling by particular modes of transport. It may even be the sight of particular people, or certain places or smells which triggers the panic, particularly in animals who have a history of being mistreated.

ROCK WATER
Mental rigidity, self-martyrdom, self-denial.

Rock Water people live life by a set of rules. Their standards are so high that they are sometimes unattainable without self-sacrifice and extreme hardship. Yet it is this very harshness and self-discipline that is the driving force of the Rock Water personality. They almost enjoy denying themselves pleasure in life, because by doing so they are reaching their goals. Rock Water people are unrelenting, and all aspects of life become dominated by self-righteousness. They may have extreme religious beliefs, or a desire to be upstanding citizens and show others by example the right way to be.

Rock Water tendencies in an animal may be difficult to detect, but they may be seen in animals that have become rigid minded in their approach to life, often as a result of human intervention. For example, there are elements of Rock Water in the military horse that is so used to being disciplined to a particular way of walking and behaving that it can no longer relax and walk and run freely. This remedy may also benefit cats that have become used to the same diet and then find it hard to become flexible and eat new things, or dogs that insist on going for walks at exactly the same hours each day, regardless of the weather or their own state of health.

SCLERANTHUS
Indecision, imbalance.
Scleranthus is the remedy for people who find it difficult to make up their minds when faced with a choice. They may find it hard to make an important decision, like who their life partner should be; or it may be a relatively trivial matter such as deciding which coat to buy. A Scleranthus type faces this dilemma all the time, but this is a remedy which can be helpful to anyone having trouble taking a decision.

The remedy is also indicated for mood swings – happy one minute, sad the next – and has been found to be helpful in other situations where balance is disturbed, such as motion sickness.

Animals, too, may display this up and down temperament. Scleranthus is seen in the cat that spends an unnecessarily long time going from one cushion to another before finally deciding which is most comfortable for settling down and falling asleep on, or in the dog that asks to go for a walk and then changes its mind as soon as you get outside.

Scleranthus animals can be unpredictable. If you are involved in show jumping, you will never be quite sure whether a Scleranthus horse will go over a particular jump with ease or refuse point blank. And as with Scleranthus humans, Scleranthus animals may suffer from mood swings and be unhappy travellers.

STAR OF BETHLEHEM
Shock.
Dr Bach described Star of Bethlehem as 'the comforter of pains and sorrows'. This is the remedy to give to those who are suffering the effects of a shocking event or accident, and to those who have received distressing news.

Any animal who has suffered shock or distress can be given Star of Bethlehem. It is one of the ingredients of Rescue Remedy which, as we shall see later, is often more readily to hand in times of crisis and may therefore be used instead. Ongoing distress, however, such as that which surrounds grief, would be more suitably assisted by the independent use of Star of Bethlehem.

Star of Bethlehem is not just for shocks that have just happened, either. Many people find it is of great benefit to animals that have suffered shocks and trauma and mistreatment in the past. For this reason many animal shelters and rescue homes use this remedy (or Rescue Remedy) on a daily basis.

SWEET CHESTNUT
Utter despair.
This is the remedy for those who have reached the end of endurance. They have suffered much, and have tried every avenue open to them, but now feel they are at breaking point and cannot see any way out of their suffering. Everything ahead is bleak and empty. Dr Bach described the Sweet Chestnut state of mind as 'the dark night of the soul' – the sufferer feels he has nothing but annihilation left to face.

This state of mind may not be immediately obvious in animals, but it is a remedy which should be considered for those who have suffered great distress and appear greatly depressed and anguished because of this. This may happen as a result of grief – for example, the dog pining for a dead master would be a suitable case for Sweet Chestnut.

VERVAIN
Overenthusiasm, a sense of injustice and the pursuit of a cause.
Vervain people feel very strongly about questions of principle and justice, and often go to great lengths to defend what they believe to be right. They will stand up for those who suffer unfair treatment and are not afraid to speak out in defence of their cause. They want others to believe as strongly as they do and will therefore invite discussion and debate as it gives them a chance to offer their point of view and put their argument forward. The intention is always to persuade others to see things the way they do – they don't want to force people to obey as Vine types do, but rather to convert them.

On a more general level, Vervain types are enthusiastic people who enjoy a challenge and will work hard at any project that they believe in. If their efforts are thwarted they become frustrated and can suffer much tension as a result.

Vervain animals are usually active and excitable and may seem highly strung. They may find it hard to keep still, and always appear interested and eager to be involved in what is going on: dogs jumping up on visitors and racing around the park to join in the ball games are Vervains.

VINE

Strong-willed dominance.

Vine people are leaders. They are strong-willed and know their own minds. They make excellent, clear-minded guides, but in their negative aspect may be inclined to use their mental strength to dominate others. In this frame of mind they can be quite ruthless, aggressive, and even cruel in their efforts to get their own way. They may ride roughshod over meeker personalities and will instruct and order other people around, expecting them to obey.

Vine animals are equally strong-minded and are keen to assume authority over the animals around them. People tend to be in awe of Vine people, and likewise, where animals are concerned, younger, small or weaker animals are in awe of the Vine, and may become nervous in his or her presence. Dominant dogs are Vine types, and unless care is taken they can assume authority over more mild-mannered human owners.

WALNUT

Protection against the influence of change.

This remedy helps those who find it difficult to adjust before, during or after a period of change. The changes in question can range from starting school to changing jobs to giving birth. Any upheaval in life which causes upset can be an indication for Walnut.

Walnut is the link-breaking remedy and will ease the transition between the past and the present. It is the remedy for those who want to move forward but find it hard to free themselves from the constraints or security of the past. Walnut is also the remedy for those who find themselves influenced by the ideas of others and are led away from their true path in life. Once again, it acts as the link-breaker, enabling progression and freedom.

For animals, the remedy would be most readily and commonly used during obvious periods of change such as birthing, being relocated during a family move, or being re-homed. It would also be helpful when another animal is added to the household, or to help deal with the changes caused by the arrival of a new baby, or of visitors or lodgers. Walnut would also be useful if you needed to leave your animal in kennels or a cattery or with friends or relatives while you are away on holiday.

WATER VIOLET
Pride, aloofness.

Water Violet people enjoy the quieter things of life. They dislike noise and disorder, and would prefer to be alone rather than be subjected to disturbance or interference. Self-sufficient, self-contained, proud and dignified, they respect other people's privacy and enjoy their own.

There is an air of serenity about Water Violet people – they keep calm in a crisis and keep their feelings to themselves. In so doing, they may bottle things up and withdraw into themselves, something which can cause them to appear aloof and unapproachable. This may increase the distance between them and other people, and instead of enjoying solitude they may begin to feel isolated and lonely.

Water Violet animals have a similar disposition. They do not complain; they rise above any problem they might have, simply wandering off quietly and alone to suffer in silence. Generally, they may appear stand-offish, and do not invite or welcome cuddles, petting or obvious affection. Nora Weeks used to say that Wumps was a Water Violet (see the Introduction).

WHITE CHESTNUT
Worrying or troublesome thoughts; mental arguments.

This remedy is helpful whenever the mind is unable to rid itself of unrelenting worrying thoughts. These are the thoughts that go round and round, that plague and pester so that no matter how interesting other activities might be the mind will be only temporarily distracted and always returns at the first opportunity to the subject of worry. This state of mind may result in insomnia, restlessness or an apparent lack of interest in what is going on around.

The White Chestnut state in animals gives rise to a similar restless state of mind. The animal may give its emotional state away by its body language or by whimpering, whinnying or crying. It may also become excessively active or agitated. This may suggest other remedies as well, but White Chestnut should be considered as a helper remedy for restless, troubled-looking animals.

WILD OAT
Lack of direction; unfulfilled ambitions.

People in the Wild Oat state of mind feel they have reached a crossroads in life. They yearn to do something worthwhile, but do not know which path to take. They may have tried several options but still feel dissatisfied with life or with their achievements. Wild Oat helps them to find direction and feel more fulfilled.

Animals may also reach the stage where they feel lost and without direction. This may happen to any animal that is suddenly uprooted from a situation in which it felt fulfilled and placed into one where its former reason for living no longer exists. Imagine for example a working dog who has been retired to a new home. He may be taken in by his owners family who do their best to make him welcome, but if his whole life has been built around his life on the farm he may feel that there is no purpose in his life any more, and feel dissatisfied and frustrated. Wild Oat is one remedy to consider, to help him rediscover a sense of purpose and fulfilment in his new home. In this situation it would probably be given along with Walnut.

WILD ROSE
Apathy; resignation.
Wild Rose is for life's drifters, people who are happy to sit back and freewheel through the years, not minding where they end up. There is no problem with this so long as the person concerned is happy – something which is generally the case with true Wild Rose types. However, there are times when people of this nature, or in this frame of mind, feel that life is passing them by, that they are missing out. They want to pull themselves out of their apathetic state but are unable to do so. Wild Rose helps them to feel more motivated and alive, so that they can get more out of life.

Wild Rose animals can be recognised by their demeanour. They tend to be mildly submissive, allowing you to do anything to them or with them, but without caring much either way. They will lack energy and enthusiasm, and only rarely get worked up or interested in anything.

WILLOW
Resentment, bitterness, self-pity.
Willow is the remedy for those who are filled with self-pity: 'poor old me' is their motto. People in the Willow state will grumble and moan about their lot in life, as though they and they alone are carrying the burden of life. If something goes wrong, it is always someone else's fault; and if someone else has some good fortune then it is always seen as undeserved.

The Willow mood is an introspective one, and by its very nature it draws the emotions down into a spiral of negativity. The remedy helps people in this state of mind to look beyond their own troubles. It lets them look at life more optimistically and recognise the positive things that it has to offer.

Animals in a similar self-pitying, tail-between-the-legs mood will also benefit from Willow. The remedy will help rid them of the depressing, resentful self-pity which causes them to mooch around and feel sorry for themselves.

RESCUE REMEDY

For emergencies and crisis situations.

Rescue Remedy is a combination of five of the 38 remedies, namely:
- Star of Bethlehem – for shock
- Rock Rose – for terror and panic
- Cherry Plum – for hysteria or loss of control
- Impatiens – for impatience and agitation, something which is often associated with pain
- Clematis – for faintness and bemused, stunned, ungrounded feelings

This combination was specifically selected by Dr Bach for all kinds of emergency situations, from shocking events like accidents, to traumatic experiences such as being attacked or receiving serious distressing news, to the thought of a forthcoming dental appointment, sitting an examination or attending an interview. In any situation that causes a person to feel shocked and terrified or nervous in the extreme, Rescue Remedy is the ideal remedy to bring instant relief.

It is frequently recommended for animals because there is so often an element of one or more Rescue Remedy indicators associated with their distress. Rescue Remedy may be used on its own or combined with one or more of the individual remedies, depending on the needs of the animal concerned. The usual method of administration is by mouth, diluted in water, but it may be applied externally if necessary. This would be a particularly useful method if the animal is unconscious or very drowsy so that it is difficult to give it orally. In such cases, moisten the lips if possible, and/or apply it to the paw pads, underside of the hooves, belly, on the nose and on the ears. These are the most delicate parts of the body and the remedy will be absorbed quickly from these areas.

Rescue Cream contains Rescue Remedy plus Crab Apple for its cleansing qualities. It is a handy way of applying Rescue Remedy externally and has been found to be extremely useful to help restore and promote the healing of wounds, bruised tissue, inflammation, and skin problems generally – in other words the external manifestations that often accompany the Rescue Remedy and/or Crab Apple states. It can be applied as liberally as necessary and may be used beneath a dressing if required. If the area is left open, it does not matter if the cream is licked as it is harmless.

Dosage

The standard dosage for animals is based on the standard instructions for humans:

A. Add two drops of each individual stock remedy to a 30 ml bottle of water. From this bottle (called a **treatment bottle**) take four drops at a time, at least four times a day.

   If you are including Rescue Remedy stock in the bottle, then add four drops of this instead of two.

B. If you prefer, or to cater for passing moods rather than deeper problems, add the same number of drops to a glass of water (for people) or a bowl of water (for cats, dogs etc.) and sip at regular intervals throughout the day.

You can mix up to six or seven remedies together, and for this purpose Rescue Remedy counts as a single remedy. Mixing in more remedies is not harmful, but the results may be disappointing: taking too many remedies together makes it more difficult for the essential remedies to do their work efficiently. It is rather like a piece of music – a fine balance of instruments creates harmony, but too much all at once is just a lot of noise. Any combination of remedies can be taken together, and even seeming opposites such as Centaury and Vine will not cancel each other out.

In humans the dosage is the same for adults and children. In the same way, when treating animals, the size of the animal is immaterial – the amount of remedy required is the same whether it is being given to a horse or a hamster. Things only get more complicated than this where there is a problem ensuring that the animal actually takes the minimum dose – in other words, the equivalent of four drops from a 30 ml treatment bottle.

For smaller animals, as long as they take a drink at least four times a day then the easiest way to give the remedies is to mix them in bowl and add more remedies every time you change the water, as in method B above. However, some animals only go to their water bowl once a day and so would not be taking the remedies regularly enough. Where this is a problem we would suggest that a treatment bottle is prepared. Doses may be given directly into the mouth from the dropper (although you need to be careful not to let the animal swallow or break the glass dropper) or via a spoon. Alternatively make up the required mix in a cup of water and then offer this solution, a spoonful at a time, at least four times a day.

Whether the mix is in a treatment bottle or a cup, you can if you want sprinkle the diluted remedies on food, as long as it will all be eaten so that the dose is taken. If this is not possible try moistening the lips with the remedies, or dripping the solution onto the nose, where the animal will lick it off. The remedies can also be applied to the pads of paws or the ears – they will either be licked off or absorbed through the skin.

For larger animals – horses, cattle, pigs etc. – the recommendation is to put the required drops from a treatment bottle on a cube of sugar, a carrot or some other acceptable snack. Again, the dosage is the same: four drops from the treatment bottle, four times a day. However, for practical reasons, it may not be possible to give remedies in this way to larger animals. The solution then is to make up a bigger version of the bowl of water that you would leave out for the cat. In order to ensure the animal takes the minimum dose even with a small drink the number of drops put in from the stock bottle should be slightly more than doubled: in other words, five drops of each individual remedy or 10 drops of Rescue Remedy per bucket of water. There is no danger of overdosing so it is generally better to give more than enough and be certain that the minimum dose has been ingested, rather than give barely enough and worry in case it has not been sufficient.

The remedies are entirely safe and harmless, so don't be afraid to experiment. You do however need to be aware of the alcohol content of the remedies.

All the remedies are bottled in 27 per cent proof brandy. If an animal is taking a medicine which is specifically contraindicated with alcohol, or if it has been found to be allergic or hypersensitive to alcohol, it may not be possible give the remedies even when highly diluted as in a treatment bottle. If you are in any doubt you should speak to your vet who will be able to offer appropriate advice and the necessary reassurance for you to do the best you can for the animal in your care.

The word 'simplicity' runs through all aspects of Dr Bach's work. He said that taking the remedies should be as natural as eating and drinking, breathing and sleeping. We know when we have had an adequate amount of sleep because we feel refreshed. We know when we have had sufficient food because we no longer feel hungry. So it is with the remedies. We know when to stop giving them because our animal patients feel better – they are themselves again.

Legal considerations for practitioners

In the United Kingdom the law on treating people with complementary medicines is extremely lax. Anyone who wants to can set up as a complementary practitioner, regardless of how much or how little training she has had, and treat people who walk in off the street. As long as she is not making unsubstantiated claims about her treatments, and as long as she does not break any other laws or injure her clients, she is free to practise.

It was partly in an attempt to set some standards in Bach Flower Remedy use amongst practitioners that the Dr Edward Bach Foundation was set up by the Bach Centre, in order to train and register practitioners under a strict Code of Practice. But not everyone offering treatment with the remedies is registered, or even trained, and this will always be the case unless and until the law changes.

It is not like this in other parts of the world, where the practice of complementary medicine is often much more difficult and in some places scarcely legal, regardless of the professional status of the practitioners involved. In some countries people cannot prepare a treatment bottle of remedies for the use of others. Instead they have to send clients along to a pharmacist who will mix up the remedies there. In other places, offering consultations is itself a problematical process that can attract the unwanted attention of the law.

It strikes many observers as bizarre that while anyone in Britain can start treating people with no need to train in anything, the law on treating animals is actually far stricter. The theory that the British love their dogs more than they love each other seems to have more than hearsay on its side...

There are numerous laws that control who can treat animals in Britain, and what they can treat them with. The situation is a complicated one. A book like this does not seek to offer legal advice, especially since the law is always open to interpretation. But based on information received from vets and other animal health professionals, and also with the help of the legal department at the Royal College of Veterinary

Surgeons, we believe we have arrived at a consensus on what is and is not allowed in the UK.

The first thing to stress is that the owner of an animal, or another member of the owner's household, *is* allowed to give it minor medical treatment. In other words, you are allowed to select and give remedies to your cat, and so are your partner and your children.

This is sensible, since giving the remedies is an entirely safe process. The genuine Bach Flower Remedies are licensed over-the-counter medicines. They have been around for 60 years and in that time it has been shown over and over again that they are harmless and safe to use. If the wrong remedy is given no harm results – picking the wrong remedy simply means that nothing will happen. So there is every reason to feel confident about trying them at home.

The situation becomes much more complicated, however, if you are treating animals that belong to someone else.

In an emergency, of course, where an animal is in pain or suffering or is dying, anyone can give minor treatment. So in an emergency you can give Rescue Remedy to the neighbour's cat while you wait for assistance from the vet. Beyond this, however, the law in the UK states that only vets are allowed to diagnose and treat medical or behavioural conditions in animals. Whether treatment of an emotional attitude or spiritual conflict should be considered to be treating a medical or behavioural condition is open to debate. Nevertheless, if a case ever came to court (to our knowledge it hasn't happened yet) it may be possible to argue that 'diagnosing' includes evaluating an animal's state of mind, so that even if you are selecting remedies for a friend's animal but leaving the friend to buy the remedies from the local shop this could be seen as treating a medical condition.

Doubtless, in everyday life people do treat their friends' animals every minute of every day of the year. And there is little chance that action will be taken against you for advising your neighbour over the garden fence to give Mimulus to a cat who is scared of going to the vet. But if you are working as a professional practitioner, and taking money for helping animals with the remedies, then you will want to be sure that nothing you do is unlawful.

The good news is that it is in fact possible to treat other people's animals, professionally or otherwise, and to obey the law at the same time. This is because you are allowed to treat an animal with the remedies as long as the vet who has charge of the animal's care has referred the animal to you. And the referral process itself is often a simple formality. It may be as straightforward as your making a telephone call to the vet's surgery so that a note can be made on the animal's file.

Under the Dr Edward Bach Foundation's Code of Practice practitioners registered with the Foundation are advised that 'in conditions requiring medical attention, the client must immediately be advised to consult with a competent licensed physician or doctor' and that 'it is the client's responsibility to take appropriate medical advice'. All the law does, in effect, is insist that these guidelines are followed for animals before they are treated.

(Remember, too, that the remedies do not treat any medical conditions directly. No practitioner should ever become involved in a situation where he or she appears to be diagnosing or treating medical conditions. Sick animals should see a vet first.)

The rather conservative approach that the law in the UK takes reflects a conservative attitude on the part of the veterinary establishment. Qualified animal behaviourists are bound by the law just as any Bach practitioner, and despite their specialist expertise they can only work with animals referred to them by a vet. And believe it or not veterinary surgeons who have qualified in complementary therapies in addition to their orthodox qualifications are also obliged to work only on animals that have been referred to them by entirely orthodox vets. In effect they are made subservient to fellow professionals who have fewer qualifications than they do.

The situation outside the UK varies widely. Within the US, for example, the law varies in severity from state to state. Because of this complexity it is difficult to offer much real guidance to practitioners outside the UK. Contact the local vet for advice, and if in doubt err on the side of caution – for example, it is probably safer to offer opinions about which remedies to choose, rather than to offer direct treatment. The Dr Edward Bach Foundation encourages its practitioners to teach clients how to use the remedies for themselves, and leaving the task of buying and mixing remedies to the individual animal carers concerned is an excellent way of achieving this.

Models for the future

We have seen that most doctors treating people are beginning to value the insights and approaches brought by the complementary school of medicine. Has the same degree of acceptance been shown by veterinarians?

The answer is a qualified 'yes'. Most individual vets are, in fact, open to different approaches, and prepared to at least give things a try. Homoeopathy, for example, is used by many vets nowadays, and if other treatments such as aromatherapy and the various forms of remedial massage are less known in the animal world this is probably as much a reflection of the way these techniques have traditionally concentrated on treating humans, as it is a criticism of the veterinary profession.

It's probably fair to say that most vets would say that they have never heard of Dr Bach or his work – until, that is, you mention Rescue Remedy. Most of them will then admit to a nodding acquaintance with the system, because even if they haven't used Rescue Remedy themselves to help calm distressed and frightened patients they will almost certainly have had (human) clients who use it on their animals.

A quick scan of the internet shows many examples of vets who have gone a great deal further, by making complementary medicine in general, and the remedies in particular, an integral part of their approach. In the UK there are complementary veterinary surgeries that offer nothing but this approach. As we have seen, the cautious attitude adopted by the establishment means that they are obliged only to work on animals referred to them by conventional vets – but the fact that such referrals happen every day shows that this route is increasingly accepted.

This is why we can be optimistic and say that we believe that in animal care as in the health care of humans, Dr Bach's work will indeed prove to be the medicine of the future.

Getting the vet on your side

Unfortunately not every vet will be as convinced of the benefits of the remedies as you might wish. In extreme situations you may find that your use of the remedies draws disbelief or even ridicule. Is there anything you can do to persuade your vet of the validity of what you are doing?

The first thing you can do, obviously, is to stress that they will not do any harm. As has been mentioned, the genuine Bach Flower Remedies are licensed medicines, produced under strict quality control, and in their 60 years of use they have never caused harm to any creature.

The second thing is to mention the many cases where they have been helpful to animals. There are many such cases scattered throughout this book, from practitioners and members of the public alike. (And incidentally, these and the many thousands of other cases we have heard about or witnessed are one reason why we can discount the argument that the remedies are simple placebos. Animals don't get better because of the power of suggestion.)

You might also stress the complementary nature of the treatment. The remedies do not replace the many skills and tools of the vet – instead they are an additional tool to place alongside them. Having read this book you will not be in a position to be your own vet, and this admission on your part should allay any suspicions to the contrary.

But the best argument, and the best way to convince any sceptic of the value of the remedies, is to demonstrate their use. Use them, and let your vet see them in action. This is how the remedies have convinced millions of people around the world that they are effective. And each person who sees you using them has the same potential to help people and animals to better health, once they too take them into their lives.

CHAPTER 3:

Reading Animal Behaviour

Principles of selection

'Many of our readers have found the Bach Remedies are most beneficial to animals, for animals have the same temperamental difficulties as we do. They may be frightened and nervous, angry, impatient, dreamy, want to be alone or continually want attention. Every cat, every dog, in fact every animal is a definite individual, with its characteristics, its own personality, so prescribing for them is simple.'

Nora Weeks, *Newsletter*, March 1968

Why is it so many actors and actresses say that you should never work with animals or children? One reason might be that animals and children are too up-front about how they feel. If they are bored by the play they will lie down and go to sleep, and if they are uncomfortable they will fidget. This is not being disobedient or wilfully disruptive, and there are no ulterior motives – they just do what comes naturally. This can make them embarrassing co-workers in a profession that relies on faking emotions.

All adult human beings are actors. We grow up learning how to suppress the way we really feel. We bite our tongues rather than give offence; we feign enthusiasm when we feel dispirited; we smile politely when we feel like murder. Over time the layers of our pretence build up, and some of us become so adept at concealment that we really have forgotten who we are. Our personalities appear entirely different from our true natures, and by the time this out of balance approach to life

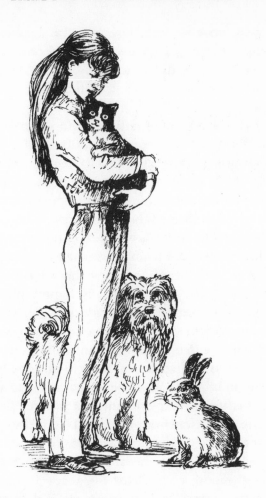

reaches full maturity there may be multiple layers of hardened emotion hiding the real person underneath.

Animals are, in general, less complex. Some may still hide their emotions, perhaps in the Agrimony way, by playing the clown when there is torture inside, or perhaps in the Water Violet way of withdrawing from companions to deal with things alone. But as a rule Water Violet and Agrimony animals are what they appear: Water Violet and Agrimony animals. They are less likely to be harbouring twenty other mental states hidden under this first layer.

If this general rule is true then selecting remedies for animals really is a simple process of empathy and understanding, as Nora Weeks rightly pointed out. Where it becomes harder is at those points where communication between species breaks down – in other words, when we misread or simply fail to read what an animal is telling us. For example, two dogs start to bark. One may be aggressive or barking in anger, and the other may bark just as loudly due to fear or excitement. How do we know the difference? How do we determine whether our dog (or cat or rabbit) is defensive and angry, or defensive and frightened?

Human beings use a mixture of verbal and non-verbal communication. So do animals. With us verbal communication is the most important system, or at least, this is generally taken to be so (although it could be argued that it is not as reliable as body language, since it is harder to deceive using the latter). With animals the opposite is true: most communication is expressed through body language. This means that to be able to select remedies for animals with real confidence we need to take time to learn a little about how animals use their bodies to communicate.

Let's imagine an actual case and how the selection process might work. Suppose your dog, who is usually happy, playful and loving towards you, suddenly begins moping around, tail between his legs, shying away whenever you show concern or affection. You know immediately from this change in manner that something is troubling him. He cannot tell you what is wrong, so you have to observe him and make a judgement based on his current behaviour pattern and apparent mood, compared with his usual temperament and nature. The first thing to note is the way he shies away from you, wants to be by himself, resisting consolation, interference or affection. This desire for solitude is a strong indicator for the Water Violet remedy. Secondly, the drooping tail gives away a depressed mood, so perhaps he needs Gentian or Gorse or Sweet Chestnut, or maybe Willow or Mustard. To determine which it is, you will need to think about what might have caused the mood in the first place. It occurs to you that he has been like this since your neighbours moved away, and you remember how well he got on with their children. You conclude that he is missing them and finding it hard to adjust. You therefore select Walnut (for the change in circumstances) and Honeysuckle (for thoughts of longing for the past) as these two remedies address the cause of the depressed mood. Water Violet addresses the individual way of dealing with it. These three remedies together would be the most appropriate personal remedy mixture for your dog.

When a practitioner selects remedies for a human client, conclusions are drawn mainly on the strength of verbal indications – body language, gesture and so on are a useful back-up to the verbal information, or an indication that more verbal information needs to be sought. With animals the order of priority is reversed. Indeed, as the example of our

Water Violet dog demonstrates, body language and behaviour alone can give all the clues that are needed.

We will look more closely at examples of body language later in this chapter. Before that, however, we haven't yet said the last word on words...

Verbal communication

Dr Doolittle could talk to the animals, and understand them when they talked to him. Sadly, the rest of us are not so fortunate. Nevertheless, we can hope to tell a little from the verbal language of animals, especially since different sounds have so much meaning for other animals: in some songbirds, for example, the song of the individual indicates not only the type of bird but also the strength of the singer, and therefore how much of a threat it would be to competitors invading its territory.

Furthermore, and at a different level of consciousness, some animals definitely do use the different sounds they make to communicate different ideas and concepts to each other. In Africa, for example, it has been shown that the vervet monkey uses two different alarm calls, one for snakes and one for eagles. When the eagle call sounds the monkeys look up and climb down; but when the snake call rings out they look to the forest floor and climb up. Clearly the sounds are associated in their minds with specific concepts. The simplest explanation for their behaviour is that they are using a language with clearly defined sound symbols for eagle-threat and snake-threat.

Mother cats have been seen to do a similar thing when bringing back prey to their kittens. They make a soft sound when they are bringing back a mouse and a harsher sound when bringing back a rat, which is a potentially dangerous animal for a young kitten. The kittens approach the prey more warily when the rat sound is made but are more devil-may-care when the mouse sound is made. Again, the different sounds are associated with different concepts, and the theory that the sounds in question are associated with 'mouse' and 'rat' rather than with, say, 'safe' and 'dangerous' is strengthened somewhat by the fact that mother cats call 'rat' even when they are only bringing in a very dead and very small piece of rat, which could be of no earthly danger to the kittens.

In 1944 a lady called Mildred Moelk did some research into the verbal language of cats and was able to separate out 16 types of sound, each with its own distinct and different meaning to other cats. Cats use their voices to signal a wide range of emotions, and with a little practice it is possible to distinguish between them and eavesdrop on the cats' conversations. It has even been suggested that some cats, with a particular aptitude for vocalising their feelings, actually build up their own personal vocabulary of vowel sounds that they use to communicate quite distinct meanings to their human guardians. It is as if over time an agreed vocabulary develops between animal and owner which allows the cat to use words to demand food, attention, or a clean litter tray.

If your cat does this you probably already know about it; even if it doesn't you can resort to the basic shared cat vocabulary to help you understand the animal's state of mind.

Basic cat sounds include the various shades of mew, spitting, hissing, and a kind of stuttering sound that usually means the cat is frustrated in some way. Some sounds are made for both people and other cats, such as the chirruping sound that mother cats make to their kittens, which is also made to their humans on occasion. In both cases it is used as a greeting, and also as an invitation to follow the chirruper. But not all of this verbal repertoire is used to communicate with us: some sounds seem reserved for other cats, such as the caterwauling and screeching of cats mating, fighting or squaring up to each other. The meaning of the long-drawn-out howls made by angry cats is one of dominance and aggression: 'stay back or else' would be a rough translation into English.

Frightened cats, on the other hand, will tend to be silent. But if cornered the frightened animal will threaten the aggressor by hissing, spitting and yowling. The sounds are similar to those of a hissing snake, which has suggested the theory that there is in fact a link: the cat is copying the sound of a feared and dangerous animal to discourage its assailants from a further attack.

The best-known cat sound is of course the purr, and it is also the one that everyone thinks they understand. Yet in fact the purr is a good example of how no one piece of body language or vocal signal always means the same thing – context is everything. Most people would interpret a purr as a signal of contentment and well-being. But in some circumstances it can be a way of inviting closer contact, for example when approaching an owner. Dominant cats might purr to an inferior cat or a kitten as a sign that this is a good time to play, so that the inferior animal can take liberties it would not normally be allowed. In the normal course of things cats in great pain will shriek, squeal, and scream; but sometimes a cat that is frightened or in pain, even one that has been severely injured or is terminally ill, will purr instead. It is as if the sound of the purr helps to keep them calm, and works as a comforting displacement activity, an attempt to soldier on bravely – the equivalent of a dying man singing a lullaby to himself or reciting poetry. One thinks immediately of Agrimony and Oak as possible remedies to give a cat in this situation.

Because of the wide range of possible meanings it has, the behaviourist Desmond Morris has compared cats when they are purring to people when they are smiling: the sound may mean that the cat is happy, but it can have lots of other meanings too. The same could be said of the mew, which is another extremely interesting sound with a number of potential meanings. Domestic cats who want attention from humans mew as they did to their mothers when they were kittens. Different tones and intensity of mew form a complete language to indicate the degree of anxiety, need or impatience attached to the basic demand for attention; these sounds vary greatly and are used to get humans to do what the cat wants. The fact that only domestic adult cats use the mew in this way is revealing because in wild cats it disappears along with the end of kittenhood.

If the vocal world of cats is a complex one, the utterances of dogs are somewhat less so, although, in practice they can be just as hard to read. Where there are at least 16 basic sounds in the cat language, there are only five in the dog's: a moaning noise, which is a pleasure sound; a howl, which is aimed at gaining something; barking and growling, which are mainly made to ward off threats; whimpering and whining, which like the mewing of cats are infantile sounds, used in this case to persuade mothers to let down milk; and the yelp, a startle sound made after a surprise or on feeling pain.

Again as with cats, some sounds are reserved for human communication. Whining is one example, as it is not usually directed at other dogs but only at humans. Dogs seem to have learned over thousands of years that whining is a good way of getting what they want from humans; howling on the other hand is aimed mainly at other dogs, and is based on the noises that wolves make to co-ordinate the pack and call it together, and to sound the alarm.

Again, the commonest sound turns out to be one of the most complex: barking can mean lots of different things. As well as the basic warning noise it can be used to communicate with humans, such as when demanding to be let into or out of the house. It can also be a sign of anxiety and even desperation. Certainly understanding the reasons why a particular dog is barking can be vital. Legal action can be taken against the owners of dogs that bark all the time; and much more importantly the animal may be in severe mental and emotional distress. The bark is its cry for help.

Non-verbal communication

As we saw earlier, vocal utterances alone are probably not going to tell you all you need to know. Unfortunately some of the other communication methods animals use will tell us even less. Of the main methods of communication used by most animals, smell is almost certainly the most important, but thanks to our infinitely inferior sense of smell it is also the one that we are least well placed to read. We don't have the equipment to appreciate the innumerable messages in urine marking, for example, and can do no more than note when the behaviour increases and try to find a reason for it – perhaps an interloper laying down a marking in your cat's territory; perhaps a change in the household upsetting your dog. When it comes to direct communication we are reduced to relying on what are probably secondary means of communication to our animals, such as expression and body language.

Fortunately body language in particular is one area that even a novice can learn to read a little. Basically, relaxed animals look relaxed; alert or tense animals hold their bodies more stiffly; and most animals with teeth to bare will bare them when they want to keep someone or something at bay. You don't need to know all about animal body language to tell the difference between two friendly dogs and two dogs who are suspicious of each other and ready to test each other out. With no particular knowledge, then, some information can be gained; and with a little study it is possible to tell a great deal more about an animal's state of mind from the things it does and the way in which it does them.

Let's look first at body language in cats. Here, at once, we find the general rule that it is possible to isolate particular areas of an animal's body that are especially likely to signal its basic state of mind. The key elements in cats are the ears, whiskers, eyes and tail, and the general body position and shape.

These elements can be thought of as words in a sentence – by themselves their messages may not be conclusive, but if several elements point in the same direction then it is fairly clear what the cat is trying to say. This is a demonstration of a second general rule that applies to all animals – and to people, come to that – the need to try to get an over-

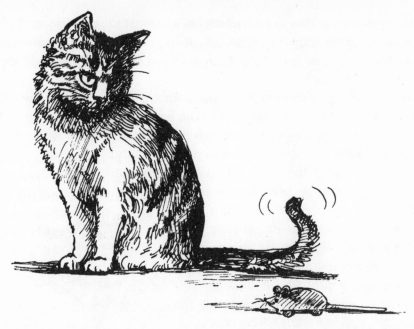

all picture. Different parts of the same animal may be sending different messages, so to rely only on what the tail says, for example, may be misleading.

If forced to choose the most expressive part of a cat's physical vocabulary one might select its delicate and sensitive ears. There are five basic positions:

1. **Relaxed:** the openings of the ears point forward and out a little; the cat is alert to any interesting sound coming from any point around about. This is the cat that is greeting someone or exploring.

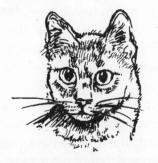

2. **Alert:** erect ears with the openings pointing straight ahead in the direction the cat is staring; the cat is concentrating on a particular sound coming from a particular point.

3. **Agitated:** the ears twitch.

4. **Defensive:** the ears are flattened back against the skull so that seen from the front they are practically invisible; the ears are vulnerable during a fight, so flattening them back is a natural thing to do if the cat fears an attack.

5. **Aggressive:** the ears are rotated back but are not completely flattened, so that from the front the back of the ears can be seen; this is a mix of the defensive position, ready to flatten back if there is an attack, and the alert position, pricked to pick up sound.

To interpret all of this into actual behaviour and remedy selection, imagine a cat that is displaying aggression. If the cat's ears stand out and can be seen from the front this tends to indicate dominance aggression, in other words an animal that wants to impose its will on another and is prepared to attack. Remedies such as Vine and Beech might be appropriate. Where the ears are more pulled down into the 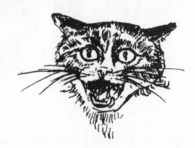 side, so that from the front you can hardly see them, then this would tend to indicate fear-based aggression, and in these circumstances remedies such as Mimulus, Rock Rose or Rescue Remedy might be more appropriate.

The position of the cat's whiskers is also a good guide to its emotional state. Fanned out and pointing forward implies attention and a state of 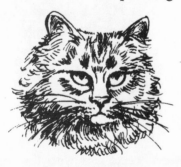 readiness – the cat may be investigating, curious or threatening; sideways and not so fanned out is the relaxed position; and the fear position is bunched up and pressed back against the face – the cat may be trying not to touch something or feeling defensive. Compare this with the forward-pointing ears of the alert cat and the fearful cat's ears pulled back snug against the skull.

Although cats do not consciously exercise control over their ears or whiskers, they do have some control. Other body signs are different in that they cannot be controlled at all, and the eyes are a good example of this. Two cats squaring up to each other can appear equally aggressive and determined, and it is only when you see that one has narrowed pupils while those of the other are fully dilated that you can tell that the first cat is the aggressor while the second is afraid and only using aggression as a means of defence.

Unfortunately the eyes are perhaps the hardest element to read in body language. Changes in pupil size caused by the amount of light or the nearness of an object can be taken, all too easily, as signs of a change in mood. If you are staring too hard at your cat's eyes, trying to read its mood, your staring will itself cause that mood to change: staring in cats signals aggressive intent, so by staring you are exerting dominance on your cat.

With this in mind, what do dilated pupils actually mean, when they don't mean too little light? The simple (and unhelpful) answer is that they mean the cat is emotionally aroused – but the actual emotions aroused can vary widely. It can be pleasure, as with a hungry cat seeing food, or displeasure, as with fear. Other elements of body language, and knowledge of the context of the behaviour, will indicate which type of emotion is actually being aroused. The one thing we can say is that if a cat's pupils are fully dilated in good light that means that the cat is peculiarly interested in what is going on.

A different form of emotional arousal is linked to contracted (closed) pupils that have been narrowed down to a slit. This means aggression and threat. If the cat with dilated pupils is reacting to an external stimulus, the cat with contracted pupils is itself a stimulus to the reactions of other cats (or people).

As well as pupil size, also look at how the eyelids are used. On a physiological level, opening and closing the eyelids is a way of controlling and responding to light levels, but it can also signal mood. Wide

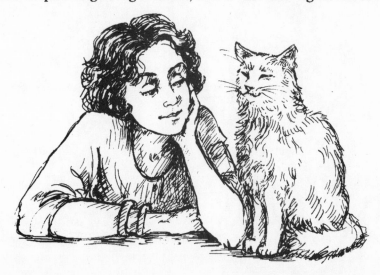

open eyes show that the cat is alert, on guard and prepared for action. Half-closed eyes mean it is relaxed and content, not feeling threatened or threatening, and trusting. Fully closed eyes (when the cat is awake!) indicate submission: this can be seen sometimes when a cat threatened by a dominant rival turns away and shuts its eyes.

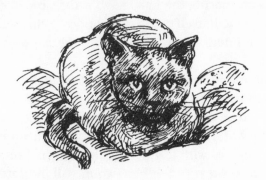

Then there is the slow, hooded blink that will be familiar to all cat owners. This has a calming effect, especially when accompanied by a long-drawn-out yawn. The message here is one of mutual recognition and reassurance. If you want to send the same message back to your cat, you could try mirroring the behaviour yourself.

Turn then to the tail. Relaxed cats hold their tails down in a relaxed curve, down from the back then up again. If the tail is held high this

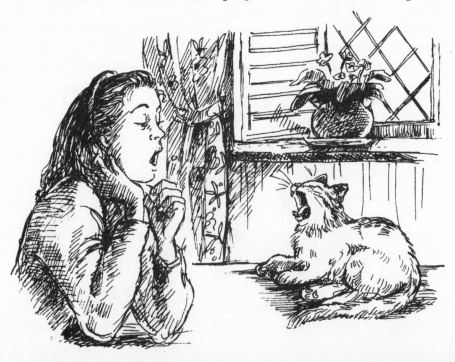

indicates a happy cat, perhaps welcoming you home – but it may also indicate other things depending on the context and other elements of body language – frustration, for example. If the tail is held high and arched over towards the backbone then this equals a very happy cat indeed.

If the tail is lowered while the tail hairs stand up then the cat is afraid and submissive; if a fluffed up tail is arched up then there is a defensive threat as well as or instead of submission – this cat may well fight rather than run. Aggressive cats who are not afraid also display a fluffed out tail, but here the tail is held stiff and straight. If the tail is arched downwards then this too may indicate aggression.

Cats will often twitch their tails from side to side when in a state of conflict, perhaps due to worry or anxiety or when they feel pulled in

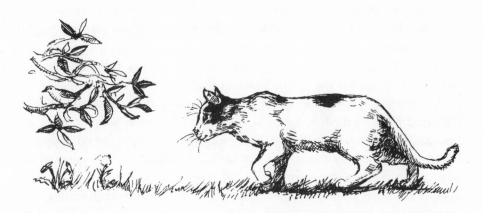

two directions by conflicting desires. Bruce Fogle gives a good example of a cat who is trying to stalk a bird across a garden lawn. In the wild, cats would attempt to catch birds from under cover. But there isn't much cover on a lawn. The cat, then, is in two minds. It wants not to be noticed – which means it will have to stay still – and it wants to catch the bird – which means it has to move forward. The tail twitches and betrays this conflict.

When the wagging is very sharp and violent, with the tail lashing from side to side, then the cat is in conflict and inclined towards aggression. And the classic 'tail between the legs' indicates submission in cats, just as it does with dogs.

Next, look at the overall posture of a cat's body. A cat with its head down and its body at a downwards angle is aggressive. If the head is held higher this shows an element of fear. Classic inter-male aggression is shown by the way two cats will stare at each other, their backs arched, approaching each other slowly.

The welcome routine of a cat performing a greeting to its human is very different. Cats demonstrating this behaviour hold their tails straight up in the air and arch up against the human. This behaviour mirrors the way kittens behave towards their mothers. Our stroking is the equivalent of the mother's grooming, and the erect tails display the anus ready for mum's inspection. The head rubbing and twining around legs is a way of marking the owner with the cat's own scent. With another cat the greeting would be head-to-head, but as we are so tall the cat makes only a token attempt to reach our heads, by rearing up slightly on its hind legs.

To sum up the two extremes of cat body language, look first at a threatening cat. Its pupils are narrowed, and this language is backed up by the head and whiskers, which are both held forward. The tail sticks straight out, perhaps with the tip turned down 90 degrees or wagging slightly. The hair along its backbone stiffens, which makes it look bigger, and its erect ears are turned around so that the backs of the ears face the threatened animal. It moves forward with its legs very straight, and with a downward slope to the front of the body.

A defensive cat, on the other hand, will have dilated pupils. Its ears flattened back against its head, it will tend to crouch low down to the floor. It, too, will have stiff hairs, but perhaps because its need to appear bigger is greater than that of a threatening animal, in this case all the hairs on its body will become erect. The body may arch up at the back, also in an effort to look bigger, and in a final attempt to discourage an attack the cat may spit or hiss.

Of course in real life not all these indications will appear together and, like people, cats can show fear in a number of ways. One reaction is to simply crouch, stay very still and not look the aggressor in the eyes. Another response is to become aggressive, approaching and then moving away from the feared thing, spitting, hissing, howling and displaying teeth and claws. And beyond pure body language, you can tell this kind of fear-based aggression from dominance aggression from the way the cat attacks. A defensive cat will tend to keep its head back away from the problem and strike out with its paws. A dominant cat will go in with its teeth, which are more formidable weapons. It is not as worried about being attacked itself.

Where there is a mix of aggression and fear there will be elements of both types of body language mixed together. For example by combining the arched back of fear with the extended legs of aggression the animal appears to be very large, an impression further strengthened by standing sideways on to the source of the threat and erecting the fur all over the body. The same mixed emotions appear for example when a cat performing a greeting holds the tip of its erect tail tilted over to one side – this shows there is some diffidence or reservation about the greeting.

There are other minor elements of the cat's body language that are worth noting. Kneading with forepaws is a sign of contentment which mirrors the action of a kitten kneading a mother when suckling. Lip-licking, on the other hand, is like a wagging tail – a sign of anxiety or conflict. Grooming is also something to watch out for. Like lip-licking, it can be a displacement activity used to release tension and calm stressed out feelings. And it is also a way of reestablishing the animal's own scent on itself, and masking other smells such as those left on a cat's fur by our affectionate stroking.

Much the same body language elements are used by dogs. The calm dog will stand with its tail and ears relaxed, and as it becomes more alert or excited so the tail and ears will gradually rise. There can be particular difficulties when breed characteristics get in the way of efficient signalling, however. Some breeds have naturally pricked ears, while others have floppy ears, and when judging the alertness of these animals you have to take the natural 'at rest' position into account.

On a dog-to-dog level, friendly behaviour includes moving along side by side, bum-sniffing, and wagging tails held at about body level. Unfriendly behaviour includes walking towards the other dog face to face with ears forward and tail arched over the back. An aggressive dog might have hackles, tail and rump all up, and it will display its teeth. Direct eye contact is also used as a means of establishing dominance, either over dogs or over people. A dog that stares you out is dominant over you, which is not a situation to be encouraged.

Dogs need to know their place in the pack, so staring out and other dominance techniques are practised at an early age between young puppies and their litter mates. Risen hackles, erect ears, bared teeth and mock mounting of rivals are all examples of behaviour that continues into adult life. Submissive puppies signal their lack of threat by lowering their heads, averting their eyes and rolling onto their backs, and this too is reflected in the way adult dogs will later behave. Other signs of submission seen in dogs of any age include the typical submissive 'grin', a grimace that does not show the teeth, and submissive urination, where a dog that is completely submissive lies down, lifts its leg and urinates.

Sometimes human beings cause this kind of submissive behaviour in dogs without meaning to. A common example is the owner who comes home to find the dog has urinated on the carpet or chewed his slippers, and stands over his dog and shouts at it. The dog refuses to look him in the eye, grins foolishly and slinks around with its head held down. The owner calls this 'guilt' and perhaps reaches for the Pine, but in fact the dog is more likely to be responding to its owner's bad mood by trying to appease him. The crawling around and so on is what the dog would do if the top dog in the pack were angry with it. The concept of 'guilt' does not attach easily to actions that to a dog would be perfectly normal, and these include such inconvenient activities as chasing cars, postmen or next-door's cat, and marking territory by urinating over your stereo. And while standing over the animal and raising your voice will clearly indicate your displeasure, the dog will not associate your anger now with its own past action. This is why dog trainers insist that the only time when a firm 'no' can be used to discourage unwanted behaviour is when the behaviour is actually taking place. Responding a second later, let alone several hours later, does not work.

Fear in dogs can manifest as overexcitement and restlessness. This might take the form of barking, or insistence on contact with the owner, or, in extreme cases, in urination and defecation. The pupils will dilate, just as they do in cats. And just as people who are nervous may yawn more or bite their nails, so dogs yawn and start to chew things. And here, once again, too much reliance on anthropomorphism can lead to errors: we might think that a dog yawning is in a Wild Rose or Hornbeam state, for example, in cases where Aspen or Mimulus might be more appropriate.

Signs of fear in dogs include the tail between the legs, crouching down, ears flattened back on the skull; and sometimes the body

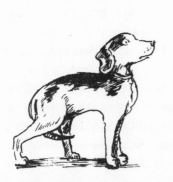
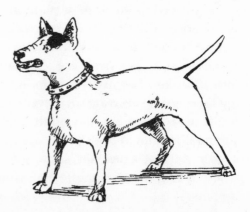

language associated with fear in dogs shows a mix that gives more information. For example, a dog with its tail between its legs (fear) and a submissive grin on its face (submission) is showing that it might know and be submissive to the person it is afraid of – probably someone in its family or pack. Another dog might have its ears plastered back against its head while at the same time it is showing some of its teeth, implying a threat. A dog like this may well bite. This reflects the fact that in many cases fear itself provokes aggression.

We have seen that both cats and dogs put their tails between their legs when they are feeling submissive. The same sort of behaviour can be seen in nervous horses who are low in the herd hierarchy. Horses also echo the behaviour of cats when faced with something they dislike or are frightened of, pulling back their heads or shying them up and away so as to avoid contact or risk of injury. And like dogs and cats, they will attack a feared person or object when escape is impossible. Indeed, any animal, even the smallest and most inoffensive, will fight to the death if there is no alternative available. And this is something we can all relate to because human beings too will instinctively pull away from something dangerous or threatening to avoid injury. And instinct fuelled by adrenalin will often provide us with the strength we never knew we had to fight an attacker. (For a more detailed examination of horse behaviour, see chapter 5.)

The parallel sign systems of different species however, do show clear differences, and some behaviour is confined entirely to only particular species. Some freshwater fish grow brighter or duller according to the amount of excitement or fear that they feel, but this insight is of no help if you want to know what a sheep is feeling. Similarly, when we humans are unsure about what to do or feel in a state of conflict, we may show it by scratching our heads or our chins. Chimpanzees also do this, or they may scratch at their arms instead – but if cats feel this way they yawn, twitch their tails or flick out their tongues to lick at their muzzles; and birds wipe their beaks on twigs.

Just as the same feelings can be demonstrated in different ways from one species to another, there are other occasions when the same behaviour can mean different things in different species. When a dog lies belly-up, for example, it is a sign of complete submission. When a cat does the same thing it may well indicate a desire to play – but the animal is actually in a position ready to attack, with the teeth and the claws of all four feet all ready for action. Cats who lie on their backs to greet their human keepers are ready to attack as soon as the play gets a little too rough for them – which is why inexperienced cat lovers often end up with their hands and arms raked raw when they make the mistake of pushing a cat over onto its back.

Despite these reservations, general sign systems based on physiological advantage can give insight into the behaviour of many different animals. Cats and dogs point their ears towards the things that interest them, and away from the things that represent a danger: the first is so that they can get as much information as possible, the second is to avoid injury. It should be no surprise to find that monkeys, horses and cattle do much the same thing. It is possible, then, to use basic knowledge of how one species behaves as a rule of thumb for other species. The insights gained in this chapter can be applied (with due caution) to the majority of the animal kingdom.

Gender differences

Knowledge of the differences between 'typical' female and male behaviour can help us define what is normal for our animals and this in turn can help us to spot the beginning of unusual mental and emotional states that might benefit from the remedies. For example, the sex of unneutered cats affects their behaviour quite dramatically. Female cats take rather more care over their personal hygiene than male cats, although they also tend to be more excitable. They are more playful than males, and are friendlier to any other cats that they live with. (The irritability shown by some mother cats is partly caused by the fact that when the kitten suckles on its mother it causes quite a lot of pain – kittens have sharp teeth, so it is no wonder that as soon as her hormone level is back to normal, a mother cat with a large litter will stop feeding them.)

Males, on the other hand, are slightly more destructive in their behaviour and slightly more active.

When we look at the difference between males that have been castrated and those that have not we find that castrated males are more hygienic and more affectionate. They like attention, and are more playful and more friendly with other cats. And males that have not been castrated are more active than their castrated brothers, which stop spraying, roaming and fighting in up to 90 per cent of cases (given that the cause of the fighting is territorial or to do with dominance – fear-based aggression and aggression against prey is not affected).

The results of neutering female cats are, as one might expect, less dramatic. It stops them ovulating and so stops mating behaviour, but that's about all. In fact, when you look for behaviour differences between neutered males and females there is very little to be found. In other words, neutering in males produces female type behaviour patterns; females, which already behave in a female way, simply go on much as before.

In dogs, there are similar differences to do with gender. For example, male dogs are more likely to be aggressive with other dogs and in defence of territory. They are marginally more likely to be playful, indulge in destructive behaviour and to be aggressive with children. On the other hand, female dogs are better at responding to obedience training, easier to house-train, and more demanding of affection.

As one might expect, and just as in cats, castration of the male dog will affect the behaviour that male dogs are more likely to engage in. So there is likely to be less aggression towards other males in castrated dogs, and they will be less likely to dominate owners and less likely to stray from home.

A specific form of aggression is linked particularly to female dogs at particular times in their fertility cycle. This is territorial or protective aggression, the kind of aggression usually shown when protecting the home, car or family, but which may also extend to the protection of favoured 'pet' objects. Protective aggression occurs in particular with female dogs following the twice-yearly surge in progesterone that prepares them for motherhood. For lack of puppies female dogs may instead adopt objects as surrogate pups, and for anything up to two months can be aggressive to anyone who tries to get hold of them. Vine might be given for particularly dominant dogs, or Chicory for those who seem unreasonably possessive, but Red Chestnut should also be considered – this is the remedy for overconcern and fear of what might happen to a loved one, and this is the anxiety at the root of the dog's seemingly irrational behaviour.

The same burst of hormones can result in depressive behaviour among bitches that can last around two months. This is the typical gloomy, motiveless depression that in Dr Bach's system is a clear indication for Mustard. This is the remedy to cast a little light and help the animal concerned to become more like its real self.

Breed differences

Just as different breeds of a single species differ in size and strength, so their emotions also will tend to differ. The more highly-bred the animal is, the more this is likely to be true, because breed animals are produced by in-breeding, and in-breeding accentuates mental traits as much as physical ones.

Breeders who selectively breed for physical characteristics such as coat colour or size are in effect favouring particular genes over others. Sometimes genes that control physical characteristics are linked to other genes that control other aspects of the animal's behaviour. When the physical gene is selected then the linked genes are also selected, and it is this principle of linkage that explains why particular breeds of animal are known to be predisposed to particular behaviour.

Linkage is not a simple thing, however. Whether mental or physical characteristics are concerned what is produced is not a cast iron characteristic but rather a tendency towards certain traits. The high number of newborn animals that professional breeders cull from every litter is a bloody reminder of how quickly and erratically new varieties of size, shape and temperament can be produced, so in the end what breeding means is that, at a genetic level, we have influenced the *amount* of *some* of its species-specific behaviours that a particular breed will *tend* to have. What we have most emphatically not done is to influence the *kind* of behaviour it will have. In other words dogs of a particular 'man-made' breed will tend to have more of some of the basic dog characteristics and less of others, but they will not have any characteristics that are outside the realms of doghood. Similarly they will tend to display more of one kind of behaviour than of another, but they will still be capable of all types of behaviour that are recognisably doggy.

In dogs which have been bred over many generations to establish entirely different body shapes, there is often a very clear link between body shape and behaviour. For example, some cocker spaniels exhibit behaviour that is graphically described by its name: the Jekyll and Hyde syndrome. This can cause them, suddenly and for no apparent reason, to fly into a rage and become aggressive, and then just as quickly become placid again. The problem seems to be linked genetically to the colour of their coats: it is most common in blond and golden cocker spaniels, less so in black ones, and those with mixed colours seem to suffer from it hardly at all. Rottweilers and Dobermanns are other breeds that can become aggressive for no apparent reason. This too may be a genetic problem and is possibly related to some kinds of epilepsy.

The link between physical and mental characteristics is less obvious in cats, which are less overbred, but it is there. If the fashion for exotic varieties continues it is likely to become more prevalent in years to come. But even at the moment it can be stated quite clearly that Oriental shorthairs like Abyssinians, Burmese and Siamese seem to be among the most outgoing, active, destructive and unbalanced of the breed cats, while Persians are on the whole more placid. Straightforward moggies, which have not been artificially selected, show more individual variation, as would be expected.

Despite the fact that purebred cats represent a very small proportion of the population, 50 per cent of cats seen by behaviourists are purebred. The reason for this may be genetic, but is also partly because they are more valuable and therefore more likely to be taken to vets and behaviourists when things go wrong. Also, breed cats are more likely to be kept indoors than others, and there are huge stress problems for a free-ranging animal when it is kept indoors in a highly artificial environment.

The link between breed and emotional characteristics applies to other animals as well. In her book *Getting in Touch with Horses*, Linda Tellington-Jones suggests a way of reading the characters of horses by interpreting the shape of their heads, ears, eyes and so on. An animal with a straight profile is uncomplicated, for example, while a double chin indicates cleverness and narrow nostrils are an indicator of a lack of mental flexibility and development. Like breed characteristics, such physical characteristics are inherited, the result of a particular mix of genes. Can they then provide a shortcut method of remedy selection?

Dr Bach once investigated a similar approach to categorising humans. In some of his earlier writings he suggested that, for example, people needing Gorse would be sallow skinned, that Water Violet people would be very straight backed, and that Impatiens types would tend to have florid complexions. He abandoned this approach when he found that it was an unreliable guide to remedy selection.

The same can be said of reading the characters of horses, or any other animals, from physical characteristics alone. Tellington-Jones is careful to say that none of the indicators she lists are to be used in isolation, and that information on the horse's general demeanour, behaviour and the kind of jobs it is asked to do are all as vital when the job of personality analysis is undertaken. As when one is treating people, then, such physical characteristics may suggest a line of enquiry, but they do not replace the empathetic job of understanding the actual emotions.

The rule that applies to horses and people applies to all animals. In the goat world, for example, Saanen goats are known for their placidity,

Anglo Nubians for their shyness (and a tendency to be bullied by other breeds), and British Alpines for their relatively wild nature. Each animal's general personality will be based on the overall genetic inheritance that has formed it, but its individuality also depends on the individual genes its parents brought to it, as opposed to the general pool of genes shared by the breed. And its personality is defined also by the way it was brought up, the things it has and has not learnt, the way it has been treated and the way it has reacted to its environment. Every individual animal is, then, more than the sum of its genes. It is an evolving, living, breathing creature. It is different from its litter mates.

What this means for us, in practice, is that in treating animals we are entitled to consider the breed in the first instance, but it should only be as a guide to the first avenue of exploration. Just as not everyone with hunched shoulders needs Gentian, just as some military policemen will be Mimulus types, so some American pit bulls will be mild, put-upon Centauries and there will be tiny lap dogs who are negative Vines through and through. Members of a particular breed might need any of the remedies at different times. All we can say of notoriously dominant breed such as rottweilers, bull terriers, akitas, chows and schnauzers is that they *tend* to be dominant and so, on average, will be more likely to be Vines or Vervains or Beeches and less likely to be Centauries, Mimuluses or Larches. But there will be many exceptions to this tendency.

You can't generalise with the remedies and, just like people, animals should always be treated as individuals and not as groups.

CHAPTER 4:

Animals in the Home

Household dogs

There are three general points worth making straight away about dogs and the way they act at home. The first is that all domestic dogs are trained dogs. We are training them all the time, whether we mean to or not – and what is more, they are training themselves. This is because whenever they do something and receive a reward they will tend to repeat the behaviour, and rewards are not all intentional.

Intentional rewards are easily understood: a pat on the head or a 'good dog' or a biscuit. Unintentional rewards are more slippery, but could be summed up as things that just happen. If your dog is frightened of your neighbour and growls at her over the garden fence so that the neighbour goes back into her house, then her disappearance is an unintentional reward. It teaches the dog that in situations where it is a bit nervous of people it's a good thing to growl because that will make them go away.

Another example is seen in those dogs that feign illness to get attention. This is probably because in the past, when they were injured, they got a response they liked. Later they will repeat the behaviour in the hope of getting the same response. There is an example of this in the Walt Disney cartoon *The Fox and the Hound*. The old dog, Chief, resents the arrival of a younger rival. Now he has broken his leg and has become the centre of attention again. He is enjoying life in the warm house, instead of being out in the wind and rain, and isn't in any real pain – but when he hears his owner return he immediately starts to howl and hobble around worse than before.

Even forms of physical punishment can be unintentional rewards because at least the animal is getting attention and physical contact of a kind from the leader of the pack. The lesson for us must be that it is important always to be careful not to inadvertently reward behaviour that we do not want to encourage.

The second general observation leads on from the above, and it is a scandal that the point still needs to be made. There is no justification whatsoever in the approach of those who say they house-train their animals by rubbing their noses in the mess. Dogs do not associate the action with the punishment – they will do so only if the two are synchronised. In other words, behaviour must be punished as it happens – if you punish a second later you are already too late and all you are doing is teaching your dog to be frightened of you.

As to the kind of punishment, only non-violent methods like surprises and reprimands should be used, and then only when absolutely necessary. Anything more, and anything too frequent, will only be counterproductive and again you will invoke nothing but fear.

Doesn't talking about training and behavioural conditioning imply seeing dogs as machines, in precisely the way we rejected in Chapter One? The answer is that conditioning doesn't exclude understanding: the salivating dogs in Pavlov's famous experiment are not demonstrating lack of consciousness but rather the opposite. They are likely to salivate on hearing the bell because they have learnt from past experience that a bell usually means food.

Finally, it is important to remember when dealing with animals that, almost invariably, they don't behave in ways we don't like in order to get even with us, or out of hatred. This is why Holly is rarely needed for animals that are behaving aggressively towards people. Instead when selecting remedies we need to look for the real cause – which is more likely to be fear, unsettlement after a change, lack of confidence and so on.

In fact, aggression caused by fear is far more common than offensive aggression, and dogs who lack self-confidence or are fearful may well turn out to be biters. Some are inclined to become overly submissive at the least sign of dominance by a human being, such as eye contact or simply standing next to the dog. They may be Mimulus types, shy and timid by nature and preferring to avoid large groups of people; or they may be Larch types – lacking in self-confidence and feeling they are not good enough; or a mixture of both. It is because they lack self-assurance that they are so ready to panic and lash out in situations that most dogs would take in their strides.

Of the actual fear remedies the most used is Mimulus, the remedy for any fear that can be named. It is good for animals afraid of thunderstorms, for example, since this is a known fear. But where the animal is actually filled with terror, so that no comfort is of use and it would run as far as it could if you let it, then Rock Rose is a better choice to overcome the panic. Where the animal appears frightened without there being any specific cause you could try Aspen, the remedy for unknown, nameless fears. Another kind of fear entirely is the fear and worry that something will happen to a loved one. Red Chestnut would be one remedy to consider for the dog who sits glued to the window pane, waiting for its human to return and becoming anxious when he or she is only a few minutes late.

Similar behaviour patterns may be evident when anxiety rather than out-and-out fear is present. With extreme or chronic anxiety, however, dogs can become neurotic and may exhibit the same type of stereotypical, repetitive behaviour that is seen in zoo animals. For example, as well as being a social exercise or simply a means to keep clean, grooming can be a way of controlling and dissipating anxiety. Rather like playing with worry beads, grooming is a comfort activity. In cases of genuine emotional distress it can become excessive and may lead to hair pulling, or licking the forelegs over and over again until the skin literally breaks down. Crab Apple would be one remedy to consider in this situation, as it is the remedy for obsessive, repetitive behaviour. But Cherry Plum would also be useful for the uncontrolled, irrational behaviour, when, seemingly, the animal doesn't know when to stop, often resulting in self injury.

It is usually much easier to help dogs who are aggressive through fear than those who simply want to be dominant. This is because fear is a learned behaviour, whereas dominance aggression has a genetic basis. The latter isn't viciousness or spite, but rather the method dogs use to define position in the pack. It happens when two dogs each want to assume the role of leader over the other – which would suggest that this kind of aggression is probably best treated with Vine.

Cases where Holly might be helpful would include situations where one animal is jealous of another. This might occur where two dogs are similar in terms of accomplishment and size, so that there is no obvious dominant one between them. They argue to find out which is which – so far a straightforward head-to-head Vine situation. But then we come along and, in trying to help defuse the confrontation, we take the side of the loser. We think of this as the humane thing to do, but for both animals it simply creates a bigger problem and in effect perpetuates the aggression existing between them. We are the leaders of the pack, and by making a fuss of the subordinant animal we are putting it into a position above the dominant one. The animal that should be dominant becomes jealous of the animal that should be subordinate, and resorts to yet more aggression to sort things out.

Giving Holly to the dominant, jealous animal should help – and the poor subordinate animal might well need Mimulus for fear of the other. But the real answer to this must be to decide which is the naturally dominant animal and then reinforce its dominance by giving it our approval. This can be done in very simple ways, such as giving that dog its food first, or greeting it first when you come home. Some might argue that this is merely pandering to the whims of the aggressor at the expense of the other animal, but the most important issue here is your dogs, and by helping them to define their social positions clearly you are responding fairly and correctly.

Urination – and especially inappropriate urination – is another behaviour that has a part to play in the demonstration of dominance and submission. In most cases it is scent marking; a dog with its leg cocked against a wall is surrounding itself with a familiar and non-threatening smell. It might be marking its territory, but in fact anxiety can be a possible cause as much as any aggressive or assertive intent. An extremely submissive dog will sometimes roll onto its back, lift its leg and urinate, and this is a sign of the utmost abandonment of any pretence at leadership. If your dog often behaves this way to you that should be a sign that you are probably rather too domineering over the animal and ought to back off a little. Give the dog Larch to increase its confidence, and think about Centaury and Mimulus as well. Vine might be a remedy to consider taking yourself.

At the other end of the feeding cycle, eating patterns can also indicate a dog's state of mind. Loss of appetite can be caused by an upset, perhaps a move to a new home or a new owner; Walnut would be the remedy to help the animal adjust to the change. Most dogs will get through this, but in some circumstances, especially where the loss of appetite has resulted in a lot of attention from the owner, the dog can actually learn to go off its food as a way of getting this attention. Here Chicory might be helpful.

Of course, there can also be physical reasons for going off food. Dogs can suffer from allergies to substances like gluten in wheat, and this is a common ingredient in some proprietary dog foods. They may appear to go off their food whereas in fact they are only trying to avoid something they are allergic to, and in this case the answer, of course, is to remove the allergen rather than rely on Bach Flower Remedies alone. Overeating can also have both physical and emotional causes, so symptoms are as likely to come from worms as from stress.

This is a general rule. Always remember that even the most obvious behavioural problem, such as scratching chairs or urinating on the carpet, may have a physical cause. Your vet will be able to put your mind at rest on this side of things while you start to look for the root cause in the animal's lifestyle and emotional state. Obsessive grooming, eating too much or not eating at all, defecating in inappropriate places – all may be a sign that the animal is under stress. But, of course, stress as a diagnosis is worth very little when it comes to selecting an appropriate remedy. What you need to do then is to look for the reason for the stress.

Animals that are very attached to their owners, for example, can suffer when they are not able to be with them. Dogs are famous for pining for dead owners or whining the weeks away when sent to holiday in kennels, but cats can go through this kind of trauma too, despite their supposed independence. In either case there are a number of remedies that could be useful: Walnut to help them adjust to the change; Honeysuckle for homesickness or for living in the past; Star of Bethlehem for shock and the sense of loss. Mimulus can also be useful, as the overriding emotion of a dog bereft of its pack leader is likely to be fear and anxiety.

Another cause of stress in dogs can be related to where you leave the animal when you are out of the house. Dogs do not necessarily prefer the wide open space of your back garden to staying indoors. Being pack animals they prefer to be where the pack is – in other words where you are. Failing that they will settle for an area that is strongly associated with the pack. So if you are out of the house, the living room, with all its smells of you and your family, is going to feel a lot safer and more relaxing than the garden where you hardly ever sit. The house is also easier to defend because it is a more enclosed territory, so there is less likelihood of the dog going frantic as might happen if it tried to preserve a large garden against every passer-by and stray cat. An ideal compromise would probably be access to a restricted outside area, with a safe bolt-hole to the inside.

You would expect Chicory type dogs to be particularly territorial, but Beech animals can be just as bad. Vervain dogs can also get over excited

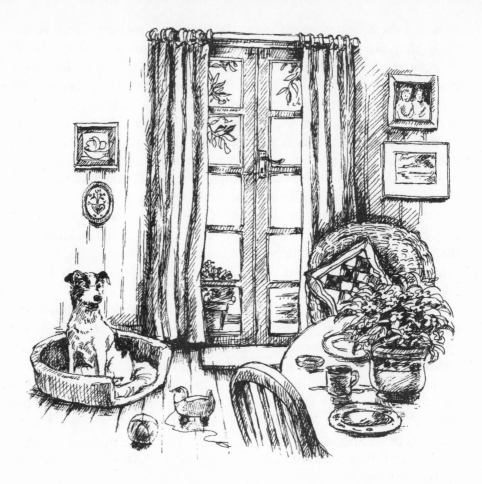

and bark very noisily in their enthusiasm for their guard duties – they can be told by the their general love of life and doggy pursuits: chasing cars and bicycles is great fun, and when not on guard they are only too pleased to leap up to welcome strangers and adopt them into the pack. Animals who lose all sense of control when left alone, to the extent where they will bite or go frantic in their efforts to escape or follow you, would benefit from Cherry Plum.

Any of the remedies can be useful, then, depending on the personality and behaviour of the individual animal. The case studies that follow demonstrate this principle and give many more examples of the remedies in action.

Dog case studies

A CASE OF NEAR STRANGULATION

Among other services I carry out, I do identification tattooing. Tattooing helps animals 'phone home' if they are lost and it helps prevent theft. It also ensures that an animal will not end up in a licensed experimental laboratory. My husband and I make the rounds of obedience classes in our area offering tattooing.

On one particular night we were tattooing a four month old akita puppy. He had just left class and was still wearing his training collar, a nylon collar which tightens when pulled.

In order to get a nice, neat tattoo, my husband Bill held the dog's back legs while the owner of the dog, in this case the husband of the couple, held the front end. I did the tattoo.

Even though the tattoo itself is painless, some animals don't like to be held in a submissive position. Every time I started to write on this particular dog he would let loose with a squirt of urine. I had to stop, mop up and begin again. After this happened several times the wife asked if she could be of help. I said yes, and handed her a wad of paper towels. She moved from the dog's head to stand between her husband and my husband so she could catch the urine.

No one realised it, but, for the whole time she was hanging on to the dog's leash. Apparently, she exerted quite a bit of force. People have heard stories about human tattoos and are sometimes apprehensive that tattooing will hurt their babies. In her nervousness she had pulled hard enough to strangle her dog.

I finished the tattoo quickly and when everyone let go we realised the puppy wasn't moving. I am a registered veterinary technician by education and I had to quickly draw on my rusty CPR training. I checked for a heartbeat. Finding none, I started external cardiac massage. This brought the heartbeat back, but no breathing was in evidence. In my distress, I forgot about the respiratory part of CPR, but as I was staring at the cyanotic (blue) gums my quick thinking husband said, 'Do you want the Rescue Remedy?'

I always have Rescue in my purse. One squirt on the dog's gums and the colour flooded back. Within a moment he took a breath. At that I gave him a second squirt (for good luck, maybe?) and gave myself one as well.

Bill and I accompanied the people and the puppy to a vet to make sure he was OK. He was given a clean bill of health. Six weeks later, when we went back to tattoo the next class, we saw the people and the dog again. There had been no problems resulting from the episode.

Betty Lewis

POST-OPERATIVE TERROR
One little dog had trauma after an operation, and for the two years that followed, was terrified when people approached him. For the past three weeks he has been on the remedies and is 80% better since. His owners are amazed.

Thank God for Dr Bach.

Judith Sanders

LIFE AT A KENNELS IN NEW HAMPSHIRE, USA
All my puppies are raised on Bach Flower Remedies. Sometimes I include information about Rescue Remedy or I place a bottle of Rescue Remedy in the puppy's care package. I also ask my puppy buyers to bring a large clean bottle with them when they come to take their puppy home. I mix Walnut for change, Star of Bethlehem for grief and separation, Mimulus for known fears and Aspen for unknown fears. I also include any remedy for that particular puppy. I fill the bottle with spring water and add the mixture for the puppy owners to take home with them. I give this to each puppy in the litter, the dam and any other of my dogs who will miss the puppy. I take the remedy myself to help me through their leaving.

One of my favourite dogs came to live with me at the age of five. He came from an area of extreme thunderstorm activity and would climb on top of me whenever there was a thunderstorm. He had other worries as well. His previous owners reported that he was frightened of cameras, loud noises and men. I administered Mimulus with great success. I realised that he was fully recovered when a very large, gruff man of the Biker variety approached while I was talking with a friend that he knew. I had completely forgotten that I had been warned that the dog was frightened of men, since he actually accepted pats from the biker.

Jeannette Nieder

LETTING GO
I use Rescue Remedy to help my animals. The cats and dogs all seem to react well to it.

One dog in particular was on the remedies a lot. She came from a rescue home, so I started her off with Star of Bethlehem and Rescue, and it just continued over the years.

She isn't with us anymore. When she was dying (a few years ago) I gave her Rescue again, along with Walnut to help her adjust to the changes. She died (she was old and sick then) but there was no pain.

From an e-mail received at the Centre

KEMO

Kemo, a three year old dog, had nervous fits ever since he was a puppy. He used to shake and shiver violently and would bark and bite other dogs and also children. His owner felt the cause was some deep-seated fear, so I gave him Mimulus, with no result, then Aspen, also with no result.

It was then that I learned he had suffered many shocks when he was a puppy, and at one time a milk truck had come to rest with its rear wheel on his head. So I gave him Star of Bethlehem.

There was tremendous improvement within a month. And after six months Kemo was a quiet, gentle, affectionate dog.

The Bach Centre Newsletter, December 1974

BRUNO – A SPECIAL HELPER

Bruno is a very special dog. He provides early warning for his master's epileptic fits. This lessens the danger by allowing prompt treatment.

Unfortunately, the dog's responsibilities make him ill. He reacts to an imminent seizure by alerting his mistress by anxious and restless behaviour. He does not settle at all until his master is back on an even keel. Sometimes this can take several days.

When his master is absent, perhaps in hospital or having day care, Bruno still knows if an episode is going to occur. Unfortunately an episode means that Bruno is ill too, with the canine equivalent of irritable bowel syndrome: he vomits daily and has very loose bowels between two and four times a day.

Rescue Remedy on its own did not settle his digestion, so I suggested adding the following remedies: Aspen for his general, vague anxiety; Chicory for his dislike of leaving his master and overprotection of 'his' humans; Crab Apple as he becomes distressed when he vomits; Mimulus for his obvious fear (just in case Aspen wasn't right); Red Chestnut as his fear is for those he cares for; and Walnut to help protect him from outside influences and to help him adjust to the changes in his household when his master is ill.

Bruno still does his job and reacts to his master's illness. However, he is much less restless and stressed and is calmer in general. His vomiting is down to about once a week instead of daily, and his bowels are much more settled. He does not cling quite so closely to his master's side.

His mistress is pleased with his improvement and gives him his remedy directly into his mouth whenever he begins to get agitated. It is also in his water bowl. There has been a steady improvement over about six weeks. We intend to continue the mixture as long as he needs it.

Clare Midgley

SEPARATION ANXIETY

This story is about a friend's Cyprus poodle, Poppy, who she rescued from ill-treatment. It constantly barked at nothing and seemed to get quite hysterical at times.

I made up a remedy of Aspen, Mimulus and Larch, having met the dog and realised how needy it was. Mimulus for its fear of being abandoned once again which manifested itself in its clingy behaviour, Aspen for its tendency to bark at things which were not there. It was full of fear. The Larch was for its lack of confidence.

According to the owner the mixture had an almost instantaneous effect, and Poppy has never reverted back to this emotional state.

Barbara Jones

BROOK

Brook is a three year old boxer bitch. She has always been a typical boxer – lively yet very friendly.

Six months ago she had her first litter of six pups. All but one of the pups were found a home and her owners decided to keep little Dave. Dave was much calmer and quieter than his mother. Brook did all the natural things you'd expect, letting Dave know who was in charge, but if Dave was given any attention she would push right in. Initially I thought it was jealousy but she didn't snap at him, she just wanted all the attention. She had also taken to escaping out of the garden, but would come back again after a matter of minutes seeking attention.

Brook had also become rather too enthusiastic with her guarding of the house. Even people she knew well were concerned about approaching. Brook could normally be walked by anybody without any problems,

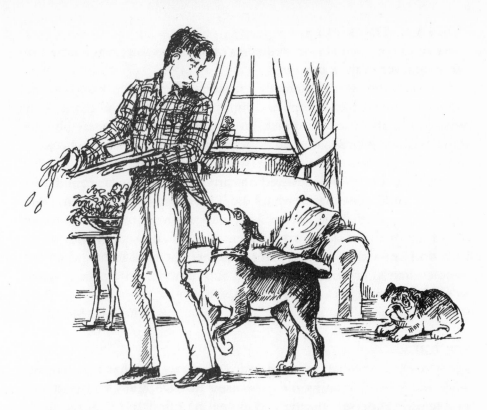

but now whether she was with her pup or not she would attack all the dogs she came across, pinning them to the ground. This was very frightening for all parties concerned, and I spoke to her owners about the Bach Remedies. Both agreed for her to have them, although one was very sceptical.

I suggested Rescue Remedy to help her with any after-effects of the birth. My second choice was Chicory for her selfish, attention-seeking behaviour. Vervain was prescribed for her overenthusiasm with guarding (and as a possible type remedy) and Beech for her intolerance of other dogs.

It was so exciting when I met her owners two weeks later and already they had a result. The sceptical partner said: 'I take it all back, it worked.' Their dog had been attacking other dogs for months, and I was told that after her first dose, she went for a walk, and though her hackles were up, there were no attacks. She was also calmer at home, allowing people at least to get to the front door before she decided whether they should be there or not, and not trying to steal all the attention her owners had to give.

Vanessa Courage

MUMS AND THEIR PUPS

I have used the Bach Flower Remedies on my dogs for a while now. I'm a firm believer in their powers.

I've used the Rescue Remedy on stressed, neonatal puppies and had what looked like a hopeless puppy come right around and start nursing. I've also used it on first time mums who were stressed by the whole birthing process. And on dogs going to their first show who were stressed by the new surroundings. Works every time.

I also had a bitch who insisted on carrying her puppies around. Just wouldn't settle in no matter what I did. I used Red Chestnut on her and kept it in her drinking water until the puppies were old enough to get out of the box. She quit carrying them around and settled with them. How do I know this was the cure? I stopped giving it to her when the puppies started creeping around and she started carrying them again. As soon as I put it back in her water she quit.

Charlotte Merrifield

SEIZURES

I have a four-and-a-half year old liver Dalmatian who has had seizures since she was 15 months old. She used to have really bad post-ictal problems, wandering, pacing and appearing blind and deaf for about an hour after a seizure. My holistic vet told me about using Rescue Remedy either to prevent a seizure, stop one or to help with the after-effects.

Since using it on an as-needed basis I have successfully stopped seizures in the middle, and now she never has any post-ictal effects. It's been a life saver for us.

Marion Mitchell

DEFUSING TENSION

I use Rescue Remedy in my dog training classes. It is GREAT for defusing stressful situations in the training room. I put a few drops in a mister and mist the room.

Lyn Richards

BELIA

Here's an animal story for you. When my small mongrel dog, Belia, was about 14 years old she became very ill. She had a high fever so I took her to the vet. He diagnosed an inflamed liver and said that it would take several days to bring her temperature down. He gave her an injection and told me I would need to bring her back for a daily injection over the next few days.

When I got her home I put a waterproof sheet and blanket on my bed and lifted her onto it. She was too ill and feeble to get up there herself. I sat beside her all that day watching TV and knitting. Every halfhour or so I would put my knitting down and wet her lips with still mineral water into which I had put some Rescue Remedy. I also put my hands gently on her to encourage healing.

She rested and slept and when she felt a bit better was able to drink some of the water from her bowl, which again had Rescue Remedy in it.

The next day she already seemed much better and when the vet took her temperature he asked me what I had done because it was right down to normal. He palpated her liver and the swelling had disappeared too. He was very interested when I told him.

Joy E. Burling

A HEATHER DOG

If I select remedies for dogs, I choose mostly a combination of three to five remedies. One time I only used Heather, for an American Staffordshire male who suffered from separation anxiety to the point that he ate himself through a 20 cm concrete wall. I gave some advice to the owners on how to treat the dog differently, as they were compensating his time alone with too much attention when they were home, and so aggravating the problem. This dog was cured in just four days.

Bianca Uittenbogaard

SOOTY

In November 1994 we received a letter asking for some help with a dog called Sooty. Sooty was 10 months old, a rescue dog, apparently given to the dogs' home because the previous owner could not cope with him.

His illness had started about five weeks before. It began with a small crust by one nostril and a slightly runny nose. He was treated with antibiotics and five days later he had become very tired and depressed, and was no better physically. A week later his nose began losing more discharge and it was suggested that he had an allergy or that he had some grass seed up his nose. He was operated on in the third week and nothing was found – but the discharge became very mucky afterwards.

A tissue analysis revealed two bacteria: staphylococci and mucoid E. coli. The condition was still not responding to antibiotics. After four weeks the vet said that it might be distemper (he had a high temperature for the first time now) and recommended that he be isolated 'just in case'.

Throughout, he ate well but was losing weight. He appeared happy and normal some of the time, like when out walking, but when he got back he immediately seemed depressed again. He had always loved company but started to hide away in dark places, and he was getting more and more tired.

Our advice was two-fold. We suggested that Sooty be given some remedies to take orally, and also that a lotion made up of Crab Apple and Rescue Remedy (or Rescue Cream) be applied to his nose. The remedies we suggested to be taken orally were:

- Rescue Remedy (to comfort him generally and help him stay calm)
- Crab Apple (as a cleanser)
- Mustard (for the bouts of depression that came and went)
- Olive (for his exhaustion)
- Oak (because he seemed to be a fighter, and this remedy would help him retain his strength)
- Agrimony (he had a happy disposition normally, and still seemed to be trying to put a brave face on things)

On 13 November, Sooty's owner wrote to us and reported: 'The first day I gave him the medicine he showed some improvement in temperament. This has been increasing daily and he's now almost as mischievous as he was two months ago.'

On 1 March the following year we heard from her again. This is what she wrote:

'Remember my dog Sooty? I thought I'd let you know that he was finally diagnosed as having a fungal condition called spongillosis at the vet hospital in Cambridge. The orthodox treatment is to drill two holes in the head and flush out his sinuses twice a day for ten days. We found a local vet willing to do this, but I insisted on waiting as Sooty had made so much progress with complementary medicine. Four vets were adamant that this could not cure him but I continued anyway. Two days ago the local vet examined and X-rayed him, and to his amazement concluded that there was no trace of the fungus. Unfortunately the sinus tissues were badly damaged but apparently this won't matter too much.'

From the Bach Centre's files

A WEST HIGHLAND TERRIER

One of my West Highland terriers had a very traumatic and serious situation recently and neither he nor I would have made it through without the remedies.

One day he was a happy, playful, joyful dog and the next he was blind and could not walk. We immediately took him to the vet, dosing him with Rescue in the meantime. The vet was happy that he was taking Rescue, and had high praise for it.

The symptoms were loss of sight and balance, and problems walking. My vet sent me to an opthamologist, thinking that there could be a vision problem. I began giving him Walnut to help him adjust to the changes, and Scleranthus for balance, as well as the Rescue.

The opthamologist ran tests that indicated the problem was neurological; we drove one and a half hours to the nearest veterinary neurologist, who put him on medication and then sent us home to watch him.

At first he seemed to improve a bit, but then he lapsed into a very serious state. He could not walk at all and was panting and shaking and appeared to be close to death.

We took him to the animal hospital, where they felt the situation was nearly hopeless and urged us to accept euthanasia. We said absolutely not; we left him overnight for tests and picked him up the next day. He was very poorly.

At home I mixed up Star of Bethlehem for the shock and trauma, with Walnut and Scleranthus as before. My state went from Red Chestnut to Gentian to Gorse to Sweet Chestnut to Star of Bethlehem – the comfort I got from that allowed me to realise that he could make it.

It is now several weeks later. It has been slow going, but he improves daily and has begun to run and jump and get excited when we get home like he always did. The Walnut has helped him adjust to his loss of sight – he is still blind in one eye – and we are continuing him on Star of Bethlehem plus Mimulus (for a fear he has developed of my husband, who carried him into the vets' offices each time) and Aspen (as he barks at shadows now, not being able to identify what they are).

The remedies helped me and my beloved dog through a terrible and heart-wrenching time and allowed all of us to have hope.

Lucille Arcouet

Household cats

For many years it was thought that cats were solitary creatures by nature who preferred a minimum of social interaction with other cats. More recently, research is tending to show that if they are left to their own devices groups of cats will interact in ways that are actually modelled very closely on what happens with lions living in pride lands: matrilineal descent, dominant males, other males challenging for dominance, and animals living together and greeting each other.

All of these things can happen in domestic cats as well, but whether or not they actually do happen seems to be dependent on the amount of food available and where the food is, and also on how many cats are living in the same area. There is also some genetic basis for differences between breeds, and of course there are the effects of interference by cat owners.

Perhaps the many misunderstandings about cat behaviour come from the fact that cats are so adaptable and subtle compared with other species. Dominance aggression in cats is less defined than in dogs, for example, in the sense that cats don't have the same sort of strict, fixed hierarchy. With cats, the dominant animal is the animal in a position of dominance at a given moment. This position can be arrived at through one cat being on its own territory, or closer to its own territory than the other cat; it can be that the two animals have met before and one animal has shown dominance over the other; or it can be simply that the cat who arrives at a particular place first is dominant. And if two cats meet like this the cat who starts off being dominant may not end up being dominant, because a cat can easily overturn an established dominance hierarchy with an action as simple as climbing onto a parked car or a chair so as to be above the other one – looking down on it literally and figuratively.

Another reason why it isn't always easy to tell which of two cats is dominant is because the dominant animal does not necessarily attack first. Sometimes subordinate cats might be first to strike, taking a quick poke at a dominant cat before retreating. A cat can also make a great show of being dominant and aggressive when really it isn't, and once the show is over the cat's place in the hierarchy is not necessarily at the top. We can also fail to notice dominant behaviour in cats because, unlike dogs they do not as a rule play dominance games with us.

The strength of social cohesion in groups of cats can be seen in the way some cats will grieve when another cat in the family dies; but others in the same situation seem to feel that a weight has been lifted from their shoulders. There are stories of cats who have blossomed following the death of a feline companion. They are usually submissive animals – Centauries or Mimulus types – who have been under pressure in the company of more outgoing companions. When the boss cat has gone the underling is free to be itself again.

Although cats are so adaptable in their social structures, it is possible to reach a point where the social structure does not work very well. A good example is in the house of a confirmed cat addict, which is overrun with cats. If there isn't enough room for subordinate cats to have their own space then real problems can occur and there can be a great increase in the number of fights and in their severity. Sometimes cats can be pushed so far down the pecking order that they become pariahs, attacked by all the other cats whenever they show their faces. In a social structure free of humans these cats would leave the territory and perhaps start to climb the ladder again somewhere else. But in a human-dominated environment this may not be an option.

As this example shows, humans interfere in the lives of cats in all kinds of ways, often with the best of motives. One form of aggression that occurs with some cats is when they are being petted and seem quite happy with that, and then suddenly become irritated and lash out or bite. The only real cure for this is to learn how much petting your cat can take, and not exceed the limits. Cats are not animals who normally enjoy close physical contact with other cats or other animals so it can be disconcerting for them if you insist on it rather too much.

All cats need their own space, even if it is only a small space, and a cat confined indoors will still find a particular corner of the room or a favourite blanket that it sees as its territory and that it will defend. Owners who find that they are threatened or even attacked by their cats, perhaps at mealtimes or when they try to take them away from a favourite armchair, are the victims of territorial aggression.

Cats who attack children, on the other hand, have normally been hurt first by the child. This is simple pain-induced aggression in which they lose patience and find it difficult to tolerate other people. Obvious remedies to think about would be Impatiens or Beech, and Cherry Plum. It could also be that the cat has been hurt in the past by a child and has become fearful of, and therefore aggressive towards other children. Mimulus would be the obvious remedy to try in these circumstances.

Apparently vicious behaviour towards other cats might actually not need treatment at all. Take the example of mother cats. As their kittens grow older the mother cat will tend to need to spend more time away from the nest. She wants the kittens to stay together and she wants them to play together. But if they play with her that can actually be a backwards step. So she can get quite impatient with them. That isn't necessarily a negative emotion because there is a positive reason for it: she wants to encourage their independence and their cohesion as a social group of kittens. Later on when the kittens are playing they can square up to each other and can again look quite aggressive. But they always seem to know their limits and usually don't go beyond them. So unless there is actually a genuine problem the mere sight of two kittens displaying apparent aggression should not in itself be a reason to reach for the remedies – although there might be a case for Walnut to help the cats get on with this stage of their life free of your interference, and you might benefit from some Chicory or Red Chestnut...

Many later problems are rooted in the earlier years of kittenhood. Kittens taken away from their mothers too early, for example, show a range of problems in later life. They are more anxious and more aggressive than other cats, and they tend to take longer to learn. Early

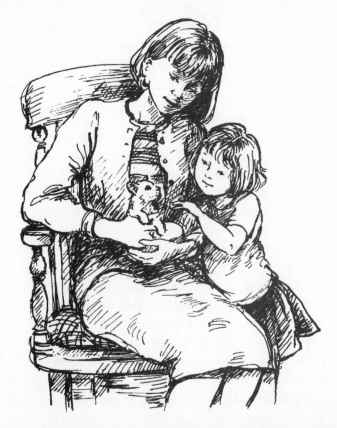

handling is vital if the cat is to be a good friend to humans, and there is research to show that handled kittens who are used to contact with humans and with other cats grow up to be more confident, more intelligent and better balanced.

Where cats are positively antisocial this may well be because they were not handled enough when they were young, and because of this they have never fully accepted people. Where they are suspicious of human beings, then Holly is a good remedy to try, along with Mimulus for fear. Other cats may become antisocial at particular times in their lives. When this happens, look for a cause. Has the cat suffered a shock of some kind? Have there been changes in its environment or home? (When they go to a new home, kittens can behave out of character for a period until they settle down, but older cats are also unsettled by a move.) Has there been an accident? Once you have pinpointed a possible cause you can begin to think about how you can help the animal to cope with it: Walnut to help adjust to changes, Star of Bethlehem for shock and so on.

If you really can't find a reason for a change of personality then it is a good idea to consult with a vet, since some physical disorders themselves can produce behavioural changes. When they are ill, some cats may become listless and irritable: they want to be left alone, they go off their food and lie around feeling sorry for themselves. In fact this is part of a cat's defence against illness: a cat loses its appetite, which means it doesn't have to go hunting, so it can save its energy to fight the infection. Fever is a good thing because it raises the body temperature and as the invading viruses usually prefer normal body temperature they cease to function as well in a body that is too hot.

On the other hand there are some diseases that cause the opposite behaviour changes. Cats become overactive, constantly wandering around; they have an insatiable appetite yet lose weight. This may well be the sign of a serious medical problem such as an overactive thyroid gland.

Cats have a better endorphin system than we do, which means that they can go about their normal business despite injuries that would have us crying in agony. They also seem far less bothered by extremes of heat and cold than we are, which is why they can sleep next to the fire and burn themselves and hardly seem to notice. This does not mean that all cats are Oak types, of course, or Rock Waters or Wild Roses, only that the thresholds for spotting these particular remedy types in cats might be higher than those we use for humans.

One aspect of cat behaviour in the home that often upsets people is what they do when they catch smaller animals and birds. This is more than just bringing prey home: it is the seemingly sadistic way in which cats will sometimes play with prey before killing it.

Research has shown that cats tend to play with prey more when they are not really sure of what to do. For example, if the animal they have caught is not one they have caught before, they will tend to play with it more than if it is something they are familiar with. They will also play with prey more when they are not really hungry or when the prey is larger than the small rodents they usually specialise in. They may simply be overexcited rather than cruel: cats like hunting, which is why they hunt, even though they are fed by us and therefore are not always hungry. They feel exuberant and excited and they display this behaviour. When the prey is subdued they can enjoy the chase without any of the danger that is sometimes attached to the prey when they first come into contact with it. They could even be scared of the prey, and although it might seem that the cat is playing with its prey as though it were a toy, the cat is actually daring itself to overcome its fear by getting closer and closer. First the cat might prod it tentatively, then roll it, then pounce on it or catch it and juggle with it, revelling in its new-found bravery. Only when the prey is sufficiently dazed will the cat position its jaws ready for a killing bite.

This is a good example then of how easy it is to misread the cat's state of mind. Playing with prey looks unnecessary and sadistic to the human observer, who would prefer a quick and more humane kill – but to the cat it is simply a sensible precaution. We also err when we speak of cats who have been told off as having their pride hurt, or going off in a sulk. Again we are misreading their reaction. In fact when they face away from their owners and sit stock-still through every rebuke they are actually avoiding eye-contact and the threat that eye-contact represents. They are not demonstrating haughtiness, but submission and fear.

This fact should also help to dispel the idea that exists even among quite experienced users of the Bach Flower Remedies, which is that all cats, or at least the vast majority of cats, are Water Violet types. Water Violet is for people and animals who are self-reliant, independent and like their own company, all attributes that are mistakenly thought of as being typical cat responses. But as we have seen, cats are social animals; far from being indifferent to others, they are just as likely as we are to become jealous when not enough attention is paid to them.

As an example, there is a cat at one of our local pubs who is in the habit of pouncing on anyone who walks in the door. It settles itself on the customer's chest, with its head in his face and forearms around his neck, and proceeds to lick his face lovingly, but very possessively. It is as though the customer has become the cat's adopted property and, understandably, he is overwhelmed by such lavish attention. This (Chicory/Heather) behaviour is about as far removed from that of a Water Violet personality as one can get.

There are Water Violet cats, of course, just as there are Water Violet people. But there are just as many Heather cats, who will demand attention from almost anyone – like the cat left at a cattery who tries to get anyone passing the cage to stay and spend time with it, regardless of whether it knows them or not. Once again, it is a mistake to generalise – you need to take each cat on its own merits, just as you would consider every human being as a unique individual.

Even more than playing with and killing prey animals, many cat lovers are driven to distraction by problems involving scent marking. Spraying or scent marking in males is predominantly a behaviour that has to do with marking out and claiming territory. Females also do it, however, and in both it can be the result of stress or of specific physical problems (in which case you need to see the vet).

Change is one real cause of stress in cats, and can hit them especially hard when they have been forced to move house. Essentially cats in this situation will tend to feel the same emotions that we do – stress, anxiety, nostalgia etc. – but it's worse for them, first because they didn't choose to move, and second because their ranges change with the change of home, and it can be difficult for them to mark out a space in a locality that up to then has been the long-established domain of the cats who were there first. In effect, they are inserted into a pre-existing territorial scheme and they have to start finding their place in that world all over again.

Walnut can be useful to ease a cat though this difficult transition, and this in turn will reduce the stress involved in moving and reduce the incidence of spraying. Mimulus might be useful, or Larch where the cat has lost its confidence and seems unwilling to go out into the garden.

Even changes that we do not think of as important can cause stress to a cat, as they have a different scale of values from ours. You might have rearranged the furniture in your living room – to the cat the heart of his territory has changed unaccountably, and he might need to reclaim it by spraying. Changes like this are the commonest cause of spraying problems.

The first clue to finding what the problem might be is to look at where the spraying is taking place. For example, if the cat is spraying up against a window that overlooks your garden it may well be that the spraying is a reaction to an event out in the garden, perhaps another cat trespassing on your cat's territory. If the spraying is caused by a particular change in the house you may well find that this will be the place where spraying will take place. And if the spraying is caused by new people arriving in the house, perhaps visitors staying the weekend or even a new baby, spraying will often be on places or objects that the cat associates with the new arrivals. Sometimes owners attribute this particular behaviour to spite on the part of the cat, or hatred, or jealousy, and so select Holly to balance that emotion. But once again the real cause is more likely to be fear and anxiety, which would indicate Mimulus, and the change itself, which would mean Walnut.

As well as using the remedies there are various other things you can do to stop a cat spraying. If a change is about to take place that you think might provoke stress you can take steps to introduce it in a measured way. For example, when moving to a new house, allow the cat to get used to one room and mark out a small territory there before giving it the challenge of defining a much larger area. If you are introducing a new cat to a house where there is already an existing cat, again keep the new one confined in a room for a few days before allowing them to meet. And if spraying is caused by the simple fact that you have too many cats in your house then consider going back to a number that can live well together in the space you have.

Cats tend to be clean animals, and in the wild will bury their own faeces – unless there is a good reason not to, such as signalling dominance to other cats. As with spraying, the first thing to do when considering a change for the worse in your cat's toilet habits is to make sure there is no physical cause, such as cystitis. Old cats, like old people, can lose control of their bladders. If this is the case the remedies can still be used alongside the vet's treatment, the aim being to keep the animal balanced, therefore giving it every chance to remain healthy and young at heart.

Once the possibility of a physical cause has been dealt with you can look at where the problem is arising to see if there is any clue there to the root cause. A new tomcat moving in next door might be enough to provoke your cat to leave its faeces unburied in your garden in an attempt to mark out its territory. In general, emotional causes for urination or defecation problems could need any of the 38 remedies, depending on the actual mental state that underlies the problem. Arguably the most common remedies involved will be Mimulus for fear, Walnut for change, Rock Rose for terror and, of course, Rescue Remedy -- but individual cats will need their own specific remedies as well.

One very practical way to help stop animals from urinating somewhere you don't want them to is to put something in the way. If your cat insists on using the corner of the living room as a toilet, block all the space with the TV or a large pot plant. By changing the geography of the space, you are forcing your cat to rethink its assumptions about where it can and can't go to the toilet.

Sometimes cats can go the opposite way and get quite fussy about where they relieve themselves. If your animal will not use its litter tray then the first thing to check is that you are keeping it clean enough. Crab Apple may help if the animal is extremely particular, refusing to use a tray that has been used by another animal, for example, or insisting that the litter be changed after every visit, no matter how minor the result.

Eating is another area where different cats will act in very different ways, and this can be one way of helping to pinpoint the animal's remedy type. Anxious cats may refuse to eat when others are around, for example, while others – perhaps with a Vine or Chicory nature – will dive in and take the best bits from all the dishes and not pay any heed to the protests of the other animals.

In the wild, cats are very successful at maintaining a healthy body shape. When cats are obese the problem almost certainly lies with the lifestyle the animal is forced to adopt, and the treatment is simple. The cat can be encouraged to lead a more active life, and you can feed it less, or feed it things that are less calorie intensive. Occasionally, however, cat owners worry that their animals are losing weight and not eating – in effect that they are becoming anorexic. This is known to happen sometimes, but it is not usually a chronic condition and the cat will start to eat again in time. Nevertheless, and to be on the safe side, where there is weight loss one should always take the animal to the vet to be sure that there is no organic cause for the problem.

Cats that are used to variety in their diet may go through phases in which they refuse to eat favourite foods. This is thought to be a survival strategy, designed to ensure that if one kind of prey is not present in the wild the cat will be able to switch to others with no problem, since it won't be hooked on one particular type of meat. There is no real problem with cats going off their favourite foods, but there can be a problem where cats are fed the same diet all the time. Eventually a monotonous diet will cause the survival strategy to fail and fall into disuse. Then if a cat is forced to change diets it can have real problems adapting. Walnut is the remedy to help adjust to changes in diet, but the real cure lies in also providing your cat with a good variety of food, and not just sticking to one or two varieties from a single make of cat food.

Cats fed a new food for the first time may scratch around the bowl and refuse to eat it. This can be interpreted as contempt or a lack of interest, but it is more likely to be a throwback to the wild, when cats scratch vegetation over a kill when they are not hungry enough to eat it now. Left alone, the cat will return to the bowl when it is hungry enough to make the new food seem palatable.

Weight loss and a refusal to eat can also be the result of stress. In that case, as always, it is important to identify the specific cause of the stress and the particular emotions that the cat is suffering from.

For example, old cats are like old people in that they like their routines to remain undisturbed. New events are not welcome and may cause some distress, and major upheavals like a change of house are especially upsetting.

Imagine then a cat living with an elderly couple. He is used to a peaceful life where he is left alone except when he wants attention, and the garden is solely his domain. This suits him fine, for he is independent and fond of his own company and pursuits. Suddenly, and to him quite out of the blue, his owners' grandchildren arrive for an extended stay. The garden is no longer his; attention is showered on him; he is pulled at and petted and chased and, of course, is under stress. He may show no obvious physical symptoms of this, or he may hide or stop eating or sit in a corner and mope, but it is the events that he needs treating for. In this case, Water Violet is the remedy for his self-sufficient nature and fondness for his own company, Walnut to help him adjust to the changes in his life and Star of Bethlehem to help him over the shock of what has happened. As usual, the emotions and the personality are treated, and the results of this approach can be amazing.

Cat case studies

NORA WEEKS ON CATS

We have had many cats, but here are three with quite different personalities and very definite ones. Catty-Cakes, a large white tom with one

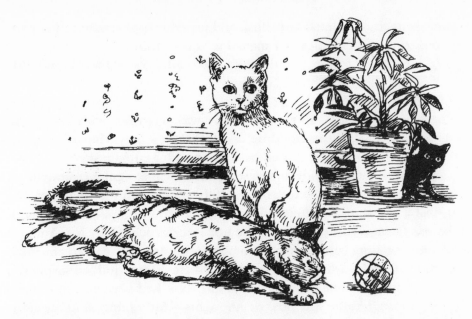

blue and one golden eye, was proud and aloof, 'the cat that walked alone' in fact. Brave, determined, uninfluenced by endearments or scolding if he wished to be about his 'lawful occasions.' A Water Violet cat, when ill he preferred to be left alone and quiet.

His wife, Lady-Love, a tabby, was quite the opposite. Affectionate, wanting to be petted, almost making herself a nuisance when visitors came, rubbing against legs. When ill, she must have attention, be stroked and spoken to. A Chicory cat.

Her son, Peggy-John, a nervous black kitten, terrified of everyone and everything. Paralysed in back legs for the first few weeks of life (Rock Rose and Centaury healed him). Hiding at first approach of visitors or any loud noise, frightened of strange cats.

Rock Rose for terror and Mimulus for his nervousness have helped him to grow into a fine strong cat, still rather nervous of strangers but able to hold his own with invading cats.

When Catty-Cakes was caught in a trap and broke a front leg, he was given his type remedy Water Violet; Crab Apple to cleanse the wound; and Impatiens and Star of Bethlehem to relieve the pain and shock. Much to his disgust, the leg was held twice a day in a jam jar containing a lotion of these remedies and the medicine was added to his drinking water – he disliked milk. The leg healed and finally he walked with no sign of a limp.

Notice whether there is fear or impatience, irritability or drowsiness, lack of strength, jealousy, restlessness, whether the animal wants to hide away or needs continual attention, and give the appropriate remedy or combination of remedies as a medicine and a lotion if necessary.

The Bach Centre Newsletter, June 1951

JENNY AND JASPER

When one of our cats, 15 year-old Jenny, was diagnosed with a stomach tumour for which little could be done, the vet's inevitable advice was that, sooner or later, we would have to consider euthanasia.

From day one of the diagnosis we gave our cat a regular treatment of Rescue Remedy to nullify the trauma of the illness and Walnut to protect against the disturbing effects of the physical and non-physical changes she was facing. We also gave her the homoeopathic remedy Nux Vom to prevent vomiting, and the essential oil of lavender was regularly burned in the room in which she slept to create a tranquil atmosphere. Throughout this time my husband and I took Red Chestnut to enable us to transmit calm and positive thoughts which Jenny undoubtedly picked up. She gradually became weaker but at no time exhibited anything more than occasional mild discomfort, still choosing to lie in a shady place outdoors and to purr loudly when approached.

One night she passed away peacefully with her head resting in my hand. The progression that her illness had taken and the manner of her passing were a triumph for this natural form of treatment. If we choose to share our lives with animals who give us great joy, we surely owe it to them, if at all possible, to say goodbye in their own time. Perhaps we should consider these natural remedies before hastening an animal's end.

The story of Jenny's passing appeared in the magazine *All About Cats* and, as a result of that article I was contacted by the owner of a cat called Jasper. He had recently been diagnosed with an inoperable pancreatic tumour. He had extreme weakness in his back legs, loss of bladder control, severe hair loss and his liver was being pushed aside to make room for the tumour to grow. She said that he spent all of his days in one room, hardly ever coming out, and that he probably only had a month or two to live.

Not wishing to raise this lady's hopes too high I explained that even where life-supporting organs were under strain or breaking down there was still no reason why, at the very least, Jasper's spirits could not be revived so that he could have a better quality of life.

I sent two treatment bottles for him which contained Crab Apple to cleanse his system, Walnut for the effects of the biological and emotional changes relating to the illness, Gorse to give him a fighting spirit, Scleranthus to help with his balance which was affected by the growing tumour and finally Rescue Remedy to address the trauma of such a chronic illness.

The day after receiving the bottles the owner rang to say that after only four doses Jasper had left his room, got up to her on his back legs for the first time, and now, as she spoke to me, he was rolling on the grass in the sunshine. About four weeks later Jasper went for more X-rays and to everyone's astonishment the tumour had gone. The vet insisted that he had not made a misdiagnosis and the owner concluded 'It must be a miracle!' She went on to say 'Jasper has really perked up no end. He was a very depressed little cat but now his character and zest for life are amazing.' She is now on the remedies herself!

Chris Newman

ZIGGY'S STORY

Ziggy, a female, eight-year-old tabby/Persian cross, was given Rock Water for her picky eating habits, Water Violet for her especially aloof nature and Vine for being the boss cat in the household, which she shared with a Labrador/setter cross.

Reported changes: her regular cat food was Sensible Choice, but the owner bought the diet version by accident because the pet store ran out of the regular brand. Generally with any food changes she would not eat for at least four days but in this instance she turned her nose up at the new food for a few hours and then ate it willingly. As a side benefit she lost the weight the owner had half-heartedly been trying to get her to lose.

Ziggy also became more active, running and playing with the dog and interacting with any visitors who came over instead of hiding or sleeping. She has also become more vocal and affectionate towards other members of the household.

Shirley Li

HARLEY

Harley, a female cat, was 13 years old when she was brought in for a consultation. Treatment was sought because she had been urinating away from her litter box. The locations she favoured were rugs and any objects closely associated with her human guardian of many years.

Discussion revealed that Harley's close feline companion had died recently, and also that her human guardian had recently married, and had merged Harley and all his possessions with his new wife's possessions and three cats, in a new home. The wife's three cats were all declawed, but Harley was not.

Since the death of her feline buddy, Harley had also been spending large amounts of time on a spot in her human guardian's bed where the deceased cat used to sleep. Often Harley would be stalked by the wife's three cats while she tried to rest in this spot.

Interestingly, Harley's guardian said that Harley would not cower or show other signs of fear or timidity when harassed by the wife's cats. In addition, Harley would show no reticence when the new wife yelled at her about her random urination. In fact, since moving into the new home, Harley would regularly climb into her guardian's lap and yap irritably at the new wife, as if trying to shoo her away if she came too near.

During the office visit, Harley was remarkably talkative and bold.

Harley's physical health was good. Though she was drinking large amounts of water, this was probably attributable to low fluid content in her diet, since recent blood tests showed no abnormalities in blood sugar or kidney function.

Harley was given the following: Star of Bethlehem for the loss of her feline companion; Honeysuckle for harking back to the time when her cat friend was alive and she had the full attention of her human; Walnut to help her adjust to the new family situation; Willow for resentment at having to share her guardian's affections; Chicory for her desire to claim and control the affections of her guardian and possess the objects she associated with him; Beech for her critical view of the new wife and the three new cats, and for the outward irritability she expressed towards them; and Larch, because I felt there was a lack of confidence at the bottom of Harley's difficulties.

Harley was given these remedies in her drinking water for a period of a month. During that time she urinated outside the litter tray only once. She seemed more comfortable with the new family situation as well. Progress was helped by environmental changes made at home, so that when things became tense between her and the other cats she could retreat to a room by herself, where she could spend time away from the other cats if she chose to.

Lucy Kaplan

A RESCUED CAT

A lady asked for help with her cat, which was terrified of its own shadow and didn't like being left on its own. She was getting desperate.

The cat's history was very sad. It had been rescued from a house where an old lady had died owning four cats. Unfortunately she wasn't found for a week and the cats had been locked in with her.

Just how badly affected this cat had been was revealed when the lady who now owned it tried to leave it in a cattery while she went on holiday. When she collected it and brought it home it yeowled for three days non-stop.

I decided to give it Rock Rose for its terror and panic at the thought of being abandoned; Star of Bethlehem for the delayed shock and trauma; and Mimulus for its fear of everyday life and its shy, retiring, nervous nature.

The lady rang a week later. There had been a dramatic improvement. Her cat had stayed out all night, which was most unusual as it normally didn't like to go out unless she went with it. Not only that but it had presented her with a live mouse the next morning (another first) – much to her dismay.

Anne Prestwich

TWO SIAMESE CATS

The female cat of this pair was suffering from cystitis and was having treatment for this with steroids and antibiotics. She was being bullied by the healthy male cat.

The owner was very caring and the house was clinically clean and tidy; the cat toys were kept in a box and the cat baskets placed at the same distance either side of the fireplace. The garden was fenced in to stop the cats from being stolen.

The male cat was given Beech for bullying. The female had Star of Bethlehem for the trauma of the tests and treatment, Gorse to lift her spirits, and Mimulus to help her come out of herself so that she could stand up to the other cat. The remedies were given in the drinking water. (I would love to have suggested Crab Apple and Chicory for the owner; what I did suggest was a shared playtime to help them all loosen up.)

After two weeks, the Beech cat was getting his comeuppance from the female and was not bullying as much. The other cat was not only more assertive, but her health was improving as well. The owner was impressed enough to buy some books on the remedies for herself. Three months further on a telephone call revealed that all was well. The two cats had regained their former friendship.

Christina Rogerson

AN AGRIMONY/CRAB APPLE CAT

Two-and-a-half years ago we adopted from the RSPCA a longhaired brown and white cat called Jasper. He had been a resident with them for over seven months. Probably the main reason he hadn't been adopted before was because he had a reputation for biting and scratching.

This didn't put us off and we brought him home. He appeared to settle very well and seemed happy and content.

But after about two weeks he started to wash and groom himself obsessively, constantly licking his back. Then he began to pull out mouthfuls of fur. In a short time his lower back and most of his tail were bald. There was no sign of any skin problem or of fleas and he continued to play and eat well.

I decided to select some remedies for him: Crab Apple for the obsessive washing and licking; Walnut to help him adjust to his new home; and Agrimony as there seemed to be some suffering underneath his very calm and contented exterior.

I gave him the remedies four times a day. Over the next two weeks he stopped pulling out his fur, although the washing continued. After a month there were signs of fur regrowth, and a few weeks later he was back to his full glossy coat.

He still scratches and bites in play, but we haven't treated this – it's just his way of having fun.

Jenny Mourant

MOMO

Last Summer our cat, who was maybe about five years old and had never been one of the fittest, stopped eating and began wasting away. The vet said he had a kidney defect, probably congenital, and wanted to put him to sleep. I felt helpless and of course the children were distressed.

To cut a long story short we decided to bring him home so that (as the children said) we could say goodbye properly. The vet did a systemic lavage and some blood tests. I have no real medical knowledge, although I have always treated my family with natural medicines: the result sheet showed a scale where his negative deficiency fell within the lower third.

We decided to treat him at home. The vet wasn't very hopeful, but she wished us luck and gave the cat a second lavage before allowing us to take him home.

We treated him with a mixture of teas, natural medicines, etherical oils and the following Bach Flower Remedies: Crab Apple, Olive, Mimulus (he was always rather easily frightened) and Chestnut Bud.

Momo recovered very quickly and after the first few days he was moving about the house again. After a little over a week he was pining to go out. We kept him on a restricted diet which wasn't very appetising for him.

Perhaps I should have continued to give him Chestnut Bud because after 10 months, just after he had been rolling around in the garden and climbing trees and I was thinking he was completely cured, he caught a bird and ate it. This is, of course, a natural thing for a cat to do. But he became sick the next day, and I knew his life was over. We had a wonderful gift of an extra 10 months. He was a happy, well loved cat and we all knew that this might happen, so were not so shocked or distressed as the first time.

Patricia Reeve-De Becker

BJ

BJ, a young, black cat I had rescued as a kitten, vomited up the entire contents of his stomach during the night. The following day he vomited up his entire breakfast several hours after consuming it. That night he vomited up a considerable amount of water. As a student of homoeopathy, my first inclination was to try out my studies. His symptoms seemed to be conspicuous by their absence, so my inexperience led me to China & Natrum muriaticum. By day four there was no sign of improvement. He was weak, dull and dehydrated (I was just able to keep him from deteriorating by giving him enemas and dripping water into his mouth).

From my experience (I have always lived in a multi-cat household), I felt he was on the way out. So I asked for help. The day I asked, your May newsletter arrived, featuring Aspen. I recalled that the reason I had rescued him was because he was so frightened. Wondering why I hadn't thought of the flower remedies sooner, I made up a bottle of Aspen, Crab Apple (to help rid him of any unwanted feelings of contamination), Hornbeam (to help him recover his strength), Olive (again for his strength), Star of Bethlehem (for the shock that must have made him frightened) and Walnut (in case he did want to move on). Aspen was undoubtedly the main remedy, in my mind.

I felt that with the first dose I gave him he would come good. The following morning (about 12 hours later) he was drinking (maybe he had during the night, while I slept). That evening (24 hours after the first dose) he was eating, albeit small amounts. Continuing with four doses a day he was back to his old, greedy self within three days. He has yet to finish his bottle of remedies, but he is absolutely back to normal now.

Thank you Edward Bach.

Madeleine Raffels

A VINE CAT

I have not treated many cats, but I have treated a Siamese cross who was very aggressive, to the point that she growled when the doorbell rang. She attacked strangers by jumping up to their faces. This cat got only Vine, and was purring to strangers within a week.

Bianca Uittenbogaard

RACHELLE

Rachelle, a 5-year-old petite tabby, was brought in for treatment of her longstanding timidity. She had been rescued from dangerous circumstances when she was already full-grown, and had never adjusted to her new home, which included three other, much more outgoing cats, a large and gentle dog, and two humans.

Rachelle spent most of her time hiding under the bed. When strangers visited she became extremely skittish, and seemed to quake, even when hiding. When she did come out she seemed to be absorbed in worry.

Rachelle was so deferential to the other animals that she would not come into the kitchen to eat until they had finished, and then she would allow the others to steal food from her plate. She never allowed herself to become involved in play. And her constant withdrawal made it difficult for her to receive any affection from her guardians.

Rachelle was given the following remedies: Aspen for her skittishness and free-floating anxieties; Mimulus for her shyness and for her specific fear of strangers and so on; White Chestnut for the mental preoccupation that her expression conveyed; Centaury for her tendency to allow herself to be taken advantage of at meals; Larch for her lack of confidence; and Walnut for her failure to adjust to her new home, even after such a long time.

Rachelle was given these remedies by dropper for a little over three weeks, at which time her guardian reported that there was some improvement. Rachelle was now coming out of her hiding places to sit next to her guardian for hours at a time, and would even hold her ground when the other cats hovered nearby. Her skittishness was somewhat reduced, and she was beginning to make gentle demands for affection. She was still quite timid, though, and if she was treated aggressively by the other cats she would roll into a tight ball. Interestingly, Rachelle's guardian believed that Rachelle felt that she deserved to be punished.

Further discussion revealed that Rachelle had spent her early years with a male litter mate who had acted as her defender. Rachelle used to imitate his behaviour and obviously admired and loved him. He was now in another home, and Rachelle's guardian seemed sure that she must miss him terribly.

Rachelle's mix was modified in the light of this new information. White Chestnut, Walnut and Centaury were dropped, and the following were added in their place: Pine for the possibility that Rachelle was not defending herself because she felt deserving of punishment; Cerato for the possibility that her early tendency to copy and seek approval from her brother contributed to her lack of assertiveness when without him; Honeysuckle for her longing for her brother; and Star of Bethlehem for the jarring effect of the separation.

After two months Rachelle was significantly bolder, even to the extent of joining the other animals for meals, and she did not allow the others to steal her food. She was spending long periods of time outside of her hiding place, and would retreat only to avoid strange visitors. Though she was still not very assertive she was more engaged in family life, and was interacting very affectionately with her guardians.

Lucy Kaplan

SPOOKY

At 14 (human) years old, our beloved Spooky was as attached to me, my husband and adult son as when he first bonded with us a kitten. Depending on his needs or mood, and our availability, he would choose one of us to attach himself to either for brushing, playing, napping or just as a paperweight when one of us was sitting at a desk to work. He always followed us around inside and outside the house, and we all enjoyed giving him the attention he wanted as he was so loving and affectionate. We, of course, were often as needy as he was.

At one point, however, we were all caught up a bit in our own lives and not able to devote as much time pampering our precious cat as he had become accustomed to. One evening I added two drops of

Chicory to his dinner after a full day of togetherness. After gobbling it all down he rushed to sit on his favourite lap to wash up and nap while I read.

He no sooner got comfortable and started cleaning himself when he looked up at me. 'What am I doing here?' he seemed to say, and quickly jumped off. He happily continued his nap in his favourite cardboard box.

I needed a little Pine after that for feeling guilty over chasing him off my lap. I also needed to assure my son that I had not changed Spooky's loving personality. Those two drops of Chicory were all that was needed to get him back into balance so that he could once again enjoy the free spirit of his feline nature.

Elisa Sampson

A STORM CAT

I became interested in the Bach Flower Remedies this summer and, after reading a couple of books, tried using them on my cat to alleviate her fears of storms. It worked very quickly and now she sits with us (rather than under the bed) and is completely calm when a storm comes. Florida, where I live, has a lot of storms so this is quite a blessing.

Judith Sanders

WHISKY

Whisky, my little, long-haired, furry, cuddly black cat, came with me to the West Indies in 1990. She had all the appropriate injections and handled the journey over to the Virgin Islands quite well. However, the weather was very hot and we both lost weight. I noticed that Whisky was fussing over her coat and constantly cleaning herself and losing fur with patches of skin emerging. The vet suggested it was hormonal and due to stress. She prescribed some drugs which seemed to accentuate the problem and antagonise her, making her attack her skin.

Whisky's personality had begun to change. She was listless, preferring to hide herself away, so I gave her Water Violet for her withdrawal and isolation, Crab Apple for her constant need to clean herself and Rescue Remedy for the stress of the move and her new surroundings.

At that time, I had to go back to England and had to leave her, along with her new remedies, for three weeks. When I returned she was a different cat. Her hair had grown back, she was not constantly biting herself and she was altogether much calmer and more easy going. The vet couldn't believe it. In fact, she took me aside and asked if the remedies worked well with children and husbands!

Ann Bruce

Other household animals

The general principles that apply to dogs and cats also apply to other common household animals, in that in all cases the key to selecting the right remedies is to try to put yourself in the position of the animal concerned.

For example, we have seen that dogs and cats are like people in that both are social animals. Relationships with others of their own kind and with humans are important to them. Most of the animals we keep as pets, such as mice, guinea pigs, rabbits and canaries, are also social animals. This simple fact can help explain the hopeless, listless behaviour of the rabbit kept in solitary confinement in a cage: try Gorse, or Sweet Chestnut, and Cherry Plum. And take advice about getting a companion for the poor animal.

Unlike cats, dogs and humans, many of the smaller animals we keep as pets are not predators but prey animals, so that a fear reaction faced with large potential aggressors like us is never far from the surface. This can be seen in the panic reactions of birds that are not used to being handled. This happens despite the fact that many birds seem to have an Agrimony type response to actual illness: they try to hide the symptoms and carry on as usual, so that only when the disease is well advanced does it become obvious. (There are good evolutionary reasons for this since in the wild sick birds attract predators and are often driven away from the safety of the flock for this very reason. Birds that can hide the symptoms of illness live longer.) But in general birds are more emotional than most other animals, which means that they may experience a great deal of stress when they come into close contact with people. Orthodox veterinary care can cause as much harm as good, with any benefits being balanced by the damage caused from handling and the application of medicines. There are cases of birds actually dying, not of disease, but of well-meant attempts to cure them. The remedies can be especially useful here, then, firstly in order to help the birds remain calm under necessary veterinary intervention, but also in order to help deal with stress in general so that stress-related medical problems do not arise in the first place.

Birds can respond particularly quickly to the remedies, perhaps because of their quick, emotional natures. But be sure to dilute the remedies before giving them to birds, as the brandy in the stock bottles can cause problems if given neat. Either place two drops of each stock remedy in the water hopper (four drops of Rescue), or make up a treatment bottle and give the drops directly from that. (See dosage instructions on page 39.)

Another typical fear reaction would be that demonstrated by the hamster that bites its loving five-year-old owner. Hamsters are simply not equipped to be dominant aggressors, but any animal that feels in fear of its life will respond by trying to defend itself – and in the wild hamsters would only be picked up in order to be eaten. Mimulus is needed for the fear, or Rock Rose for terror, or Rescue Remedy – and not Vine or Holly. Cherry Plum could be used to help overcome any tendency to lose control and lash out; and it can also be used for self-destructive stereotypical behaviour, such as repeated gnawing of limbs or plucking out of fur or feathers.

Small animal case studies

TWO RABBITS

The rabbits I treated were both dying. One was a tame Angora Rabbit, turned loose on the heather. When it was brought to me I went to the vet with it. He said it could die or live, I just had to wait and see. I put Rescue Remedy in the water bowl, but the rabbit was still lying flat on its side 24 hours later. It was wounded from a dog bite, and bled from the mouth, and from wounds on the back and genitals.

After 24 hours I realised I should have put the remedy in its mouth as it wasn't drinking by itself (this was years ago; I know better now). So I gave the remedy with a teaspoon and left the rabbit alone. His tongue was out of his mouth and it was already turning blue. Half an hour later when I checked, it had eaten and was sitting straight up, grooming itself.

The other rabbit I treated belongs to my daughter. One night it wouldn't eat and for this rabbit that was a sure sign that it was very ill indeed. As I checked it out, it had muscle tension and was very cold. When I took its temperature it turned out to be only 36° C, about two and a half degrees lower than normal. Tongue and mouth were blue. I gave it Rescue Remedy and went to the vet.

I arrived there about 20 minutes after administering the remedy.

The vet couldn't find anything wrong. And to this day the rabbit is still very healthy.

Bianca Uittenbogaard

SOME GOLDFISH

My wife changed the water in our fish bowl yesterday morning. Being in a hurry she inadvertently got the water at the wrong temperature, throwing the goldfish into shock. When we eventually noticed them they were lying on their sides near the top of the bowl apparently near death. They were lying quite still with only sporadic movement of their gills.

We put several drops of Rescue Remedy in the water although I thought it was much too late to do anything for them. Within an hour they had completely recovered. I spoke on the telephone to the lady who handles the goldfish at the pet shop, and she assures me that it is almost unheard of for goldfish to survive from the state of shock I described.

The Bach Centre Newsletter, April 1975

MORE FISH

Recently, when we had the really bad icy cold days, two of our largest fish, which reside in a garden pond, needed some emergency help. Basically I saved their lives with, of all things, mouth to mouth resuscitation and the Rescue Remedy.

On bringing the goldfish from a frozen pond, seemingly dead, and with no response after several minutes in an enamel bath, I exercised their lower chests and underbody areas trying to bring air into their bodies. For what seemed ages nothing at all was felt as I tenderly massaged each fish, holding them immersed in the water because they were almost solid and lifeless. My wife then suggested Rescue Remedy and first of all we fed two droplets into each mouth.

I repeated the massage for a few more minutes when I saw movement of a gill, then one fin twitched. We fed them two more drops of the Rescue Remedy and kept breathing into their mouths.

It was not many more minutes before we saw the smaller fish tremble, twitch and very slowly turn vertical and begin to breath unaided. The larger fish took a bit longer, but that too suddenly shuddered and trembled, and its body began to expand and contract.

I considered the recovery of the fish important enough to warrant a letter to our local newspaper, which they duly published. This created such an interest that from one article in our local press, we were on television – I did three live broadcasts – and the story went nationwide and appeared in the majority of the national papers.

J.E. Day

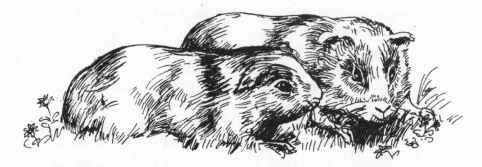

TOLLI THE GUINEA PIG

I treated our guinea pig several times. His name was Tolli and he was a male. His little companion was a female called Mini. After years of being a very lucky male guinea pig his little wife died and he was very sad. He became apathetic, didn't eat (believe me, this was very unusual for him) and he didn't make any noises (he 'talked' to my daughter every day).

I decided to give him a homoeopathic remedy, Ignatia C30, one globule, and four drops of Rescue Remedy in his drinking water. The next day all was gone – no longer apathetic and so on. He was still looking for his little wife, he was searching, but in a better mental and physical condition. In every exhausting situation after that (car driving, visit at the animal doctor, illness), I always gave him Rescue and in every case he felt fine afterwards. Now he is gone at the age of eight lucky years.

Britta Cierniak

Treating the owners

Animals have long been used to help human beings recover from illness. At the York Retreat in 1792 animal companionship was used to help treat mental patients, for example, and during the second world war patients at the US Army's hospital at Pawling in New York worked at keeping livestock as part of their therapy programme. Throughout Europe there are scores of examples of riding projects, where children and adults with mental and physical disabilities are encouraged to ride horses in order to improve their mobility, balance and self-awareness.

Dogs are given to wheelchair-bound people on the grounds that they are surer and more reliable friends than humans. And of course the commonest uses of this kind are the guide dogs for the blind programmes that operate in various countries around the world.

Animals help people, and one reason they are so good at doing this is that they empathise with us. And there may be even more to it that that: research has been done in France into whether dogs can literally smell emotion. The belief is that if people feel happy or sad or excited they will smell differently. So dogs (and presumably other animals as well) might be able to sniff out our states of mind – a thing that would allow them to become first rate Bach practitioners...

Whether this theory is true or not, what is certain is that the way we behave (our body language, our tone of voice, our personalities in general) affects the way our animals behave. Professional trainers always say that in order to teach animals well we need to start by knowing ourselves, and in particular to stay calm and aware of our own emotions. In a similar way, when selecting remedies for animals it is best to know what emotions we are feeling and, of course, to use the remedies to balance them if necessary, so that we are not reading our own out-of-balance feelings into the animal we are trying to help.

An even bigger danger of not using the remedies ourselves is that we may actually be the direct cause of our animal's negative emotional states. People in conflict are more likely to be inconsistent in the way they treat their animals and, in turn, this can cause conflict in the animal's mind. People who are frightened or anxious of something are likely to imprint anxiety onto their animals. Dogs in particular are very open to our behaviour and inclined to mimic it. There is a very strong argument for treating the dog owner before the dog. Fear in a dog, for example, may indicate that the owner is fearful and perhaps in need of help from Mimulus or Aspen.

Imagine the following scenario: a dog seems to be very demanding of attention and is always under your feet trying to attract attention to itself. When you return home it displays excessive greeting behaviour. When you go out and leave the dog behind, even for a short time, it rips into the furniture, biting and tearing the cushions and chairs and generally makes a real nuisance of itself. It really is a bad dog because you always make a special fuss of it when you have time, much more so than the other members of your family do, so it ought to be grateful.

The first thing you might be tempted to do is to give the dog Chicory for its manipulative and possessive nature, and Holly for the spiteful attack on your soft furnishings, which is obviously launched out of a desire for revenge. But the first thing you *ought* to do is look at things from the animal's point of view to be sure that the problem doesn't originate with you.

Perhaps the fuss you make of the dog from time to time is encouraging an over-strong attachment in him. What happens is that whenever that very strong attachment is threatened, even by something as simple as your going out for a walk, then the dog becomes very anxious. This triggers all the typical behaviour responses associated with animals suffering from separation anxiety, such as self-mutilation, destruction of property, inappropriate urination and barking. Rather than trying to get its own back by destroying property, anxiety is the real root cause – the animal is afraid of being deserted by the person who has made it emotionally dependent. Mimulus would be a good remedy for the dog, and while Chicory might be helpful for the animal that has been forced into this state, the creature who really needs Chicory is you.

Weight problems also tend to start with the owners rather than with the animals. Left to their own devices cats do not tend to get fat. But if they are kept in groups rather than living on their own, as happens in many households, they tend to eat more. And if they are on hormones like progesterone, which is sometimes used to treat behaviour disorders, then one side effect of these hormones is to increase appetite. Tranquillizers like diazepam (for example Valium) have a similar effect. And the other major cause of over eating in cats is boredom. People who keep their cats indoors are creating this specific problem. Their cats are inactive, they are bored, and just as we do, when they are bored they tend to eat more.

The problems – and guilt – of owners can be reflected in the problems of the pets. A dog owner who goes out to work every day may overfeed the animal out of guilt and this, plus irregular exercise, soon help it to become overweight and out of condition. Pine for guilt, and perhaps Vervain or Elm or Oak for the overwork, should be given to the owner rather than the animal.

Certainly a lot of the behavioural problems owners notice are not behavioural problems at all. They are perfectly normal behaviour patterns, but they are happening in places and in contexts that are not convenient for humans. Perhaps this is one of the reasons why the reported incidence of such problems has gone up hand in hand with the fashion for keeping pets in the house and not allowing them outside. Once upon a time cats were free to live as cats out in the big wide world and would come home when they wanted feeding, a place of refuge, or human companionship. Now they can't be cats because they are stuck indoors all the time.

In this situation there is a remedy for the owner who is overanxious about the safety of a beloved pet, and that is Red Chestnut. The cat condemned to an unnaturally sheltered life needs you to take this remedy just as much as it needs to take remedies itself.

In the same way, most animals regarded as stubborn or wilful are in fact far more likely to be confused, stressed or fearful – and the fault is likely to lie with the person whose commands are being ignored. Dogs or horses that are slow to train may be feeling fearful or stressed, and it has been shown that animals learn less, and learn more slowly, when they are under stress. Again, start by looking at your own state of mind and make sure that you yourself are not causing problems with your irritability or lack of patience. If you are calm, the animal will be calmer too, and you might find training is quicker and less of an ordeal.

CHAPTER 5:

Horses

Horse and horse

By nature, horses are affectionate and co-operative, living in communities or herds. They are naturally gregarious so suffer much from loneliness if kept in isolation. Communities in the wild generally consist of groups of about half a dozen horses – one stallion, his mares and their off-spring. Groups of stallions don't usually get on well and one stallion will fiercely see off another who tries to poach a mare or invade his family. This even happens when a male foal of the group grows up – the stallion will make it clear that the colt is no longer welcome and will forcibly evict him if necessary. Young fillies may also leave the group, but they tend to drift away of their own accord rather than be actively forced out like colts.

Sometimes a lone, family-free stallion will decide to challenge the authority of an established herd stallion and make a concerted effort to move in and take over his group of females. Usually the old, established male wins, but naturally a time will come when he will succumb to the strength and vigour of a strong, young challenger.

This behaviour among stallions, the fact that they lead their herd and aggressively protect the others, along with their willingness to fight and stand up to other stallions, may lead to the conclusion that all success-ful stallions must be Vine types. This, of course, is not true. Some may be Vines certainly, but many of them have a far more caring and pro-tective manner. If a herd takes off or flees, for example, it is usually one of the mares that leads the way, or a curious foal. The rest of the group follow and the stallion takes up the rear, making sure that they are not being pursued, and checking that none of the youngsters have been left behind. Successful stallions show strength, but in a gentle, caring way, and are tremendously resilient, ensuring safety at all times and constantly working hard to ward off possible danger. These characteristics may be true of Oak and Elm types and doubtless there are plenty of Oak stallions about. Chicory is another remedy which may apply, characterised by the possessive concern the stallion has for his mares and foals. He certainly won't share them with another male if he can help it. And of course positive Vine characteristics may be demonstrated too, such as organisational skills and the ability to shepherd and guide others.

There is no discrete subgroup of remedies that applies to all stallions, however, just as there is no subgroup of remedies for particular breeds of dog. The key, as always, is to look at the individual animal. Negative Centaury or Mimulus stallions will be unlikely to be the lead males in herds, but given the right circumstances and an absence of effective competition from other males it could happen.

Horses that are stabled where they can see other horses, while happy to have some companionship, may still fret at being kept apart from their friends. This may cause them to be quite vocal – neighing, shaking their heads or whinnying constantly – which may be a sign of their sense of insecurity at not being in more natural, open surroundings with those they know. This kind of problem may occur particularly with younger horses. Walnut may be a help for animals that have been moved from a different stable or that are being stabled for the first time. Mimulus would be for their anxiety, or Rock Rose where there is real terror. Some horses may injure themselves or lose control – Cherry Plum can be a help here. In time and with patience most horses will learn to cope with periods of aloneness and unfamiliarity, but of course the best answer would be to recreate a more natural environment for the animal. That is why, wherever possible, horses should be allowed to live out in fields, and in groups that mimic the organisation of herds in the wild. In particular, they should not be left on their own.

Given the choice, horses always prefer to set up a special pair bond with another animal. This isn't a sexual bond, but rather a friendship bond that lasts for life; if there are no other horses available the pair bond can even be with another type of animal completely, such as a donkey or goat. Pair-bonded horses look out for each other and so feel more secure. The ideal, then, would be to have an even number of animals kept together in a field – one horse by itself will feel desperately lonely, while three horses will include one that has not been able to make up a pair bond.

Like many other wild animals, the horse's sense of hearing is sensitive and highly evolved. It is there as a means of self-protection, alerting them to the threat of danger and enabling them to prepare for a fast getaway. In addition, and again as we saw earlier with dogs and cats, the position of the ears is used to signal the mood. Loosely upward with openings forward in a north easterly and north westerly direction is the neutral position. Ears rotate towards sound, so a horse interested in what is going on and picking up and taking in the important signals its surroundings give off has ears that are constantly, but smoothly, on the move, turning towards the sounds it hears. Horses are alert to their surroundings, their ears pointing ready to pick up on any danger, curiosity or friendly visitor. If an unusual sound is heard the ears will turn to listen more carefully and the horse's mind will be more focussed on the possible implications. If it is concerned it will prick up its ears even more acutely and turn its head as well, or even move its whole body to face forward so that it is in the 'ready for action' position.

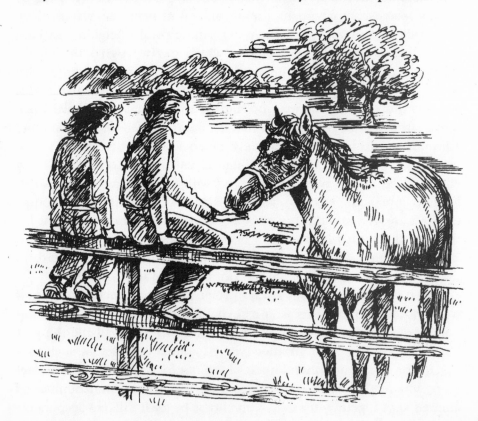

Ears that are held laterally to the head, openings pointing towards the ground, indicate that the horse is submissive, fatigued, listless or subservient, or lacks confidence. Terror and panic are identified by twitching, flicking ears. This shows that the animal is alert and ready to take flight. On the other hand, ears flattened backwards portray anger and aggression and say 'don't argue with me'. This can be seen regularly on dominant horses that like to show any newcomers who is the boss.

Tail position is also meaningful. A tail held high is a sign of alertness and vitality. One held low indicates lethargy, fear, ill health, pain or exhaustion, or is a sign of submission. A tail swishing from side to side is the horse's way of showing that he is irritated, annoyed or frustrated, and the harder it swishes and bashes, the more bad-tempered and angry the horse is – unless of course he is just swishing away flies.

Aggression is also displayed by thrusting the head or nudging with the nose. But gentle nose nudging, with the mouth closed, is a friendly way of asking for attention.

Repeated and persistent movement from the neck may signal that the horse is bored and needs stimulation or a broader environment or the company of other horses. This sign needs to be taken seriously because it can mean that the horse is going through an emotional crisis.

Generally, an elevated body posture with head held high and tail erect means the horse is excited, eager and alert. It is a sign of assertiveness, confidence and dominance. On the other hand, a sagging body, low head and limp tail, indicate boredom and drowsiness and are signs of submission.

Another sign of frustration and fear is when a horse paws the ground, scraping with one front hoof. Lifting the front leg is a warning gesture that the horse might rear up and strike with both legs – clearly a sign of annoyance, but likely to be caused by fear more often than by dominance aggression. Similarly, lifting the back leg is a defensive threat. Stamping is evidence of a threatening mood: the horse is protesting at something, and is using the stamping of its hooves to show its annoyance.

As with humans, facial expression is another revealing means of communication. Friendliness is shown by reciprocal grooming between horses, both using a similar mouth movement to gently nibble each other. This is similar to the movement used by a foal to demonstrate its submissiveness. An adult horse with wide open lips and exposed teeth, on the other hand, is threatening to bite. This teeth-baring display may also be indicative of nervousness or pain. However, this expression shouldn't be confused with the curling back of the upper lip to show the top set of teeth, accompanied by an outstretched neck, which is used by stallions aroused by the smell of a female's urine. Flared nostrils indicate excitement and keenness.

A horse's facial expression can be read easily, and, in many ways, horse expressions mirror expressions on our own faces. Closed eyes indicate the horse is either exhausted or in pain; half-closed eyes mean he is relaxed; wide open eyes indicate apprehension or fear; and looking backwards may be a sign of anger, but may also mean that something has caught the horse's interest.

It is especially important to be aware of these signals and what they mean when a mare is in foal. This is naturally a time when the horse is at its most sensitive. Mares will seek out a dark, damp place in which to give birth, somewhere that is private and away from other members of the herd. Stabled horses are, of course, limited in this respect, but nevertheless prefer to give birth at night when it is quiet and there is more privacy. Mares can control labour to a certain extent, so they can consciously wait until it is dark or until they are on their own; they do not want onlookers, a wish that we can surely sympathise with. It is painful enough being in labour, but to be a spectacle as well is bound to be more traumatic. How much more relaxed and comforting it would be to give birth in subdued lighting, and only have those people there who can add to the atmosphere and encourage you.

Before labour actually begins the mare displays agitated behaviour. She may appear restless and anxious, scraping the ground with her hooves, sweating and moving around in anticipation. She may even kick her abdomen, irritated at the growing pain and sense of tautness.

Once the foal has been delivered an important bonding process follows. This involves the mother cleaning her foal by licking off the gestational membranes and fluid. This helps her to become familiar with her foal's smell, which is not only vital in the bonding process, but also enables her to identify her foal and tell it apart from others, even in the dark. Once established, mother/foal relationships within the herd are particularly strong and may override other group hierarchies that already exist. For example a mare which, by its behaviour, is characteristically Beech with other horses in the herd, may take on strong Centaury characteristics within this particular relationship.

Suckling begins straight away, as soon as the foal has scrambled to its feet, and continues for about a year, until the mare gives birth again. At this point the first-born is rejected in favour of the youngster. This coincides with the point at which the stallion in the group, if there is one, shoos away the young males.

Horse and rider

Horses are perhaps the best example of wild animals being tamed for the purpose of living with, relating to and/or serving human beings. Every horse, no matter from what stock it has come, has to be tamed when a human being mounts its back for the first time. Its natural desire to buck and throw the rider off is schooled out of it during the process known as breaking in. The wildness, if you like, is tamed out of it. The rider is showing the horse who is in control and is teaching it to obey.

How is this likely to feel for the horse? Does the person breaking in the horse care so long as the horse becomes manageable and suitable for riding? The truth is that he or she certainly should care, because there has to be a certain rapport between horse and rider for the process to work. If there is no mutual understanding the horse will not tolerate the attempts of the rider and the rider will fail repeatedly, no matter how hard or for how long he or she tries. So who is really in control? The rider might like to think he is, but in fact both sides have to agree to work together for a successful partnership to form.

Learning to ride a horse can be usefully contrasted with learning to ride a bike. When you get on a bike for the first time you are likely to feel nervous and afraid of falling off. But once your initial nervousness has been overcome your confidence begins to rise – until the bike seems to take over, wobbles uncontrollably, and you end up on the ground. It is your own state of mind that has caused the problem because you forgot to know your own limits and go at the right speed.

Horses are a lot bigger than bikes. They have minds of their own and can actively throw you off. They feel all the emotions you do – so apprehension, fear, confusion or annoyance can make things go wrong from their side just as well as from yours. And in addition their state of mind will respond to yours – if you are diffident and indecisive the horse will lose confidence in you and will be less likely to co-operate. As far as possible, then, you have to be clear, concise, firm and know what you are doing.

Our body language shows our state of mind – round shoulders indicate someone who is fed up, depressed, tired, self-pitying or down in the dumps in some way. Moods can be almost manufactured simply by adopting the posture associated with the mood. Sit or stand round-shouldered, slump, put on a gloomy facial expression, sigh heavily, and you will soon begin to feel your spirits diminish. You no longer feel happy, buoyant or full of energy. Suddenly you feel flat. That's the effect simple body posture can have on your state of mind.

Turn this principle on its head and the reverse is true. An upright, positive, open body posture immediately makes you feel good.

Now take this onto horseback. Think about how a horse will react to a rigid, tense, anxious rider, and conversely, how it will react to a relaxed and confident one. Horses sense our demeanour and respond accordingly, so the more positively we can present ourselves, the more positive the mood and behaviour of our horse will be. As part of this positive attitude it is vital to develop trust between horse and rider – neither of you will relax if you do not trust each other.

To be trusted you need to be yourself. If you can project a sense of inner self-confidence and freedom and pleasure you and the horse will enjoy each other's company more. Walnut may well be an extremely helpful remedy here if you feel that old habits or other people's ideas on horses and on riding are stopping you from being yourself. Other remedies to consider are Cerato if you find yourself asking other people's advice when deep down you know what is right for you, Larch if you lack self-confidence, Centaury if you find it hard to assert yourself, and Mimulus to allay fear and nervousness.

The need to be yourself will apply throughout your riding career, but is harder to achieve in the early stages when learning. After all, it is difficult to give your horse the impression that you are relaxed, positive and in full control when you are a nervous and uncertain beginner. You may not realise that you are gripping too tightly with your knees or that you are pulling inconsistently on the reins, or that you are too relaxed or not relaxed enough. Fortunately there are enough calm, dependable horses around that are aware of our human shortcomings and have the good sense to ignore them. Thanks to their efforts it is possible for new riders to get through these early stages successfully.

Other horses seem less tractable and seem unwilling to tolerate beginners. When presented with a rider who clearly knows nothing they will either eject her from the saddle or refuse to move at all. Could these horses perhaps be more assertive and fiery than their more placid fellows? Are they Vine, Vervain, Impatiens or Beech types, as opposed to Oak, Elm, Centaury, Wild Rose, Agrimony or Clematis?

Perhaps; but there is an alternative explanation. As we have seen, the moods of horses can reflect the moods of riders. Otherwise confident

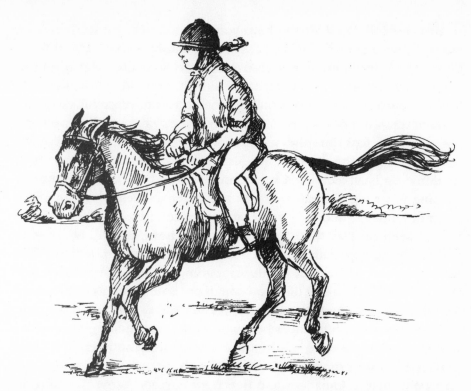

horses can become anxious when the rider is nervous or uncomfortable. When a horse receives conflicting instructions or is asked to do something unexpectedly, or is frightened by the rider's abrupt reaction, it is likely to feel afraid, or at best confused. The skittish or stubborn behaviour perceived by the rider is more likely to be based on anxiety and fear than on dominance or a stubborn refusal to obey: the conclusion is often Mimulus or Rock Rose rather than Vine or Beech.

Horses are prey animals – they are eaten by animals like us – and the relationship between our two species is coloured by this fact. In general, then, we can say that whereas Vine and the other 'strong' remedies will apply to relationships between horses, they are less likely to apply when it comes to the feelings a horse has towards its rider. Even the strongest and most dominant horse is in a subservient position to its rider. If it seems agitated, wilful, restless, stubborn or belligerent with you it is more likely to be feeling fear and desperation than hatred or superiority. And when things go wrong within this relationship the most likely candidate for Vine and Holly is you, not the horse.

For this reason it can be very useful when trying to select type remedies for a horse to see it interacting with other horses, rather than relying entirely on how it acts with people.

You certainly need all the help you can get, because deciding, for example, whether your horse's easy-going nature is that of Wild Rose, Centaury or Agrimony is not always easy. To someone who does not know the horse at all it is likely to be almost impossible to tell the difference. But careful observation will enable you to place his character more accurately. For example, Agrimony horses pretend all is well and try to avoid a fuss, but also tend to be restless. You may observe the horse scratching the ground with his hooves or tossing his head when he thinks he is all alone, yet when you are with him he acts as though nothing is wrong. Centaury horses are eager to please you and, like Agrimony horses, adopt a 'peace at any price' attitude. They tend to be less keen on play than Agrimony horses, however, and are quieter without being especially nervous – and they are always obedient. Wild Rose horses are likely to be docile, easy going, unhurried creatures, and they too prefer a fuss-free life. However, there is no particular enthusiasm for good times, as with Agrimony, or for service, as with Centaury.

There are clear differences between these three remedy types, then, and they can be used to tell one horse apart from another. The same applies to other groups of remedies that, superficially, have much in common, such as Impatiens and Beech, or Elm and Larch. The similarities may be confusing to someone meeting a horse for the first time, or to someone coming to the remedies for the first time, but with a little thought and study the owner can go a long way.

Study of your horse's personality should ideally begin before you actually buy it. Your own natural anxiety with a horse you do not know may make this difficult, but you can at least attempt to get an overview of what the horse is like before you commit yourself to a long-term relationship with it. You need to consider, among other things, its background, where and how it has been living, and whether it has been neglected in any way or has met with a trauma. These factors will help you to understand its emotional state a little better. They will also help you to forecast how many and what kind of behavioural difficulties you might have to deal with. This isn't to say that you should only take on horses that don't have any problems and come from safe, comfortable backgrounds – but if you are going to help a horse with problems then you owe it to the horse to be sure that you are in a position to offer that help, and that means anticipating the problems you might have to deal with.

It is not only the horse's previous environment that is important. Its previous rider will also have had an effect on its disposition, and if it has been used to the same rider for a long time its temperament may have become moulded and fixed hard by that rider's attitude. If the rider has been consistently fair and firm then the horse is likely to know where it stands, and there should not be too many problems. But if the previous rider has been inconsistent or temperamental then the horse too is likely to be erratic and unsure of itself. Similarly, a horse may seem rebellious or be exceptionally timid and nervous if it has been mistreated in the past – Star of Bethlehem could be useful here to help it deal with the after-effects of any trauma.

Like children, some horses may need a certain amount of behaviour training in order to help them fit into the life they have to lead. The key to good training (like the key to good parenting) is to be firm, fair and, above all, consistent. Give praise for good work and avoid confrontations by refusing to respond to tantrums. In most cases the horse will soon understand exactly where he stands, which will give him a greater sense of security and lead to more peace of mind and greater stability for both of you. The key to this has to be mutual respect.

Remedies that may help at this time include Aspen, Mimulus and Rock Rose, as appropriate, to help reduce fear and anxiety. Beech will help if your horse seems intolerant of its new home or routine and always wants to do things its own way. Honeysuckle would be a consideration for homesickness if the horse has been with a previous owner for a long time, and of course Walnut is one of the most important remedies during a period of unsettling change and will help your horse to adjust to its new home, its new environment – and to you.

By using the remedies and following a sensible and humane pro-gramme of acclimatisation your horse will gradually gain confidence and feel secure. But as we have seen already it is equally important for you to feel confident, as horses will pick up on any uncertainty, fear or negativity in your mind. A positive attitude on your part will generate more positive feelings in your horse. It will respond more readily to your commands, will gain confidence and begin to forget its feelings of insecurity. This means using the remedies yourself and so taking charge of your own state of mind and emotions.

So think about how you feel when you ride – are you afraid? Do you think your horse should obey you without question? Do you try to assume complete control? Are you made impatient or irritated by your horse's slow responses? Do you give up easily? Do you resent your horse for not performing as you would expect? There are remedies for every negative state that you might be in, and they will help you to be yourself and achieve a state of relaxed inner certainty that will make you a better rider.

Occasionally, and despite every effort, a horse may seem as though it will never settle, so that despite much positive perseverance and all the patience (and Walnut) you can muster, you come to the conclusion that you are simply not compatible. This is not defeatism, and you shouldn't feel that you have failed. Just as people are on different wavelengths – we instantly get on with some people we meet, and never feel quite comfortable with others – so sometimes we have to accept that an instant rapport, or lack of it, exists in our equine relationships.

Injury and emergencies

As we have seen, horses are sometimes labelled stubborn or wilful by their owners when fear and confusion would be a better description of their actual states of mind. These emotions can reach crisis point when the frustrated rider tries to use force to bend the animal to her will. Dr Bach put together the Rescue Remedy formula knowing it would contain something for every living creature that was faced with an emergency and filled with terror, confusion or loss of self-control as a result. That these are the emotions most often felt by animals when things go wrong is reflected in the fact that Rescue Remedy is the single most used remedy when helping animals.

Rescue Remedy can be useful in all kinds of situations. Most of us are only too aware of how stressful dental appointments can be, and of how one bad experience can colour our view of the journey to the dentist's surgery ever afterwards. For horses, shoeing can be equally stressful. Rescue Remedy – and lots of reassurance – has been found to help to instil calm and reduce the effects of fear and panic.

Similarly, Rescue Remedy can be given to help ease the shock and emotional trauma that result from an accident. It can also be applied externally to help ease the trauma associated with physical injuries and bruises. (And, of course, you should also consult the vet in such circumstances, as other treatments may be necessary as well.) Wounds tend to heal quickly in younger horses, but even here you need to watch out for fine particles of dust, grain, soil or wood as these can hinder the healing process if they get into the wound, no matter how young and fit the horse is. Keep wounds clean, adding Rescue Remedy and Crab Apple to the cleaning solution, and using Rescue Cream on and around the affected area.

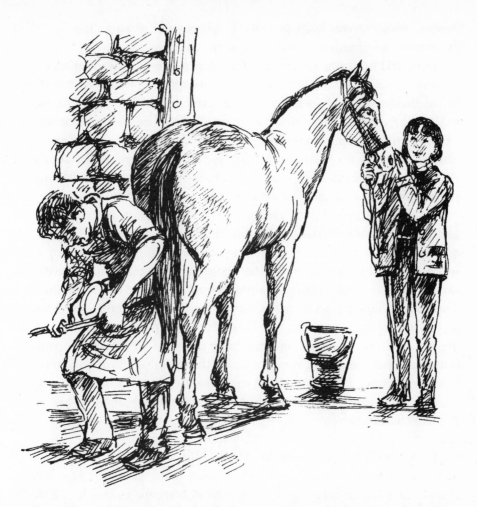

Pain due to an injury, physical strain or over exertion can sometimes give rise to symptoms that mimic behavioural problems. If you have a horse that bucks, barges and rears when an attempt is made to get him to do something, then the first thing to do is to check there are no physical problems such as back pain or other discomfort. The only way your horse can tell you if it hurts him to carry you on his back is to rear up and, if you persist, he will throw you off. It would be wise to seek professional assistance as a first resort. Once you know the cause, you can treat it appropriately.

Chomping at the bit is usually a sign of tension, a result of pain or discomfort. But it may also be emotional in origin, and indicate frustration, irritation, intolerance or annoyance. Once again seek to establish the cause and if it is emotional treat it with the appropriate remedies. If it is a physical problem this will need direct attention, but the use of

Rescue Remedy will help to relieve the mental tension that physical discomfort so often creates. This in turn will help your horse cope with the pain and be more accepting of attempts to treat and help him.

Whilst Rescue Remedy is ideal for emergency situations when the horse shows signs of shock, panic or terror, other remedies would be more appropriate where more specific states of mind are present. For example, the pain may make him feel irritable, frightened, anxious, wary, hostile, suspicious or bad-tempered. By choosing appropriate remedies you will be able to help ease your horse's discomfort indirectly by relieving the mental tension which inevitably exacerbates the pain.

As for purely emotional reasons for stress, the horse's environmental and social needs are vital considerations. Our own husbandry can minimise the horse's stress by providing the kind of environment that he will enjoy, and in which he will feel content and relaxed. We have seen how horses are naturally herd animals and therefore need companionship to live happily. An obvious way in which we can help our horse to feel at home, then, is to provide him with a companion. Of course owning two or more horses may not be a practical or affordable option, but an alternative solution might be to think about sharing stables and fields with other horse owners. There may be several of you who are in a similar situation and this would enable all of you – and your horses – to help each other.

From stable to show-ring

Horses like to have freedom, so if you are trying to stable a foal be prepared for a protest. It will be used to the closeness and reassuring contact of its mother and to the open field, so it is not surprising that it will object to being made to stay in a confined space. The fight to get out will be partly to do with fright (Mimulus, Aspen, Rock Rose) and partly to do with anger and a sense of sheer injustice (Vervain). Unfortunately, sometimes there are no alternatives to stabling for horses, for all kinds of economic, practical and social reasons; if you have to put your horses in stables they will get used to it given time and patience, but it is important to try and make the period of adjustment as comfortable and stress-free as possible.

A similar principle applies to horses who do not go into horse-boxes easily. If a foal feels claustrophobic in a stable, imagine what it must be like for a fully grown horse to have to spend any length of time in an area barely big enough to turn round in. And, of course, if he has had a previous bad experience associated with the horse-box, he is especially likely to protest next time you try to put him in – Star of Bethlehem might be useful if there is a past shock involved.

Much patience, goading and forward planning is necessary to try and foresee these problems; do whatever you can in a practical sense to minimise or overcome them. For example, don't leave everything until the last minute – make sure you allow plenty of time so that you can be calm and patient and unhurried. This will automatically transmit greater calm to your horse – far better than a flustered rider, pushed for time, ordering her panic-stricken horse into the box and both becoming increasingly agitated and upset.

Often, using the horse-box means you are on your way to a competition of some kind, and your own state of mind on the morning of a show or gymkhana may not be all it should be. Certainly, the whole environment is likely to be disrupted by the hustle and bustle of getting ready. The emotion of the occasion is so easily transmitted to the horse who in turn starts to feel anxious and tense, just at the time when you want him to be calm. On such occasions it is even more important to plan ahead and leave plenty of time; and plan to reach for the remedies when your temper starts to rise – taking them yourself at such times can be as great a help to your horse as giving him the remedies himself.

Once in the box and on the move, the horse may again feel unsettled, travel sick, frightened and panicky. Good remedies to try here are Scleranthus for the imbalance associated with motion, Mimulus and/or Aspen for the fear, and Rock Rose and Cherry Plum (or Rescue Remedy) for the different degrees of panic and loss of control.

At the show-ring itself, the nervousness of the rider can once again be harder to control than the apprehension of the horse. Competing can certainly be a nerve-wracking experience, at least in the beginning. Rescue Remedy is the most suitable remedy for competition nerves – for both you and your horse. Vervain can be helpful if you (or the horse) are overexcited or full of pent-up energy and overeager to get out there; and Impatiens if you are inclined to be too quick-thinking for your own good – making assumptions too soon, trying to get the horse to jump or turn before he is ready, and generally lacking patience.

Because the remedies are so gentle and non-intrusive you can trust them to help you and your horse make the journey from stable to show ring in as calm and relaxed a way as possible. You will both arrive in a better frame of mind, able to enjoy the event together without unnecessary angst and worry.

Horse case histories

THE DANGER OF NETTLES

Whilst staying with my friend, we decided to take our dogs out for a run. We were about to leave when there was knock on the door. It was a young girl, very agitated, saying that she had come across a horse that had collapsed in the lane nearby. The horse's rider had sent the girl to get help.

My friend offered to call the vet but the girl said the rider needed help now. It was Sunday afternoon and we were miles away from the nearest vet's surgery. I always carry Rescue Remedy with me so I ran to where the girl said the horse was, taking my friend with me as she is used to handling horses and I'm not. When we arrived the horse was on her feet but leaning into the hedge. She was totally rigid and seemed unable to move at all, except for her eyes which were rolling and showing the whites. She felt extremely hot, she was sweating and there were large bumps and weals on her chest, flanks, neck and front legs. Worst of all her tongue was very swollen and protruding from her mouth with her teeth embedded in it, making it difficult for her to breathe.

Her rider was very shocked and upset – tearful, having an asthma attack, close to vomiting – but she refused the Rescue Remedy when I offered it to her. Despite her distress she was able to tell me that Mitzie (the horse) had just cantered through some nettles and had also eaten some. She'd then bucked and reared, collapsed, managed to get up again but then was unable to move at all.

Mitzie was now aged four; she had suffered an allergic reaction to nettles when she was a foal and, at the time, the vet had diagnosed anaphylactic shock, but this had been forgotten about until now.

I really thought the horse was going to die. I thought the Rescue Remedy might just save her, or at least allow her to die peacefully and unafraid. With her rider's permission I rubbed the drops onto Mitzie's tongue and gums, and within less than one minute her eyes stopped rolling and she gazed calmly at me. I rubbed in more drops and her muscles began to relax and she was able to stand up properly. Her tongue was shrinking rapidly and her breathing was back to normal. I continued to give doses of Rescue Remedy every few minutes, and within a few more minutes she could walk and had cooled down considerably. The bumps and weals (nettle rash) were diminishing fast.

Within about 15 minutes of our arrival on the scene Mitzie was back to normal, apart from slight remnants of the nettle rash and a slight cut on her foot, sustained when she was rearing. She and her rider were able to walk the three or four miles home without difficulty. I gave the rider, Karen, the remains of the bottle of Rescue Remedy and advised her to add it to some cool water to bathe the area affected by the rash when she got home. I also gave her my phone number so she could let me know how Mitzie was.

When I got home there was a message on my answerphone from Karen to say that she had got home without any further problem and had completed Mitzie's treatment by bathing her with the Rescue Remedy as advised. The remains of the nettle rash had gone and Mitzie was back to her usual self. I don't know much about horses or allergic reactions (and the beauty of these remedies is that you don't have to), but I do feel that Dr Bach's Rescue Remedy might just have saved Mitzie's life.

From a registered practitioner

GOLDIE

AMERICA. Mrs A. Ferguson of Santa Cruz, California has been treating the mare, Goldie. On 13 October her owners noticed for the first time that she was blind. There was a white half-moon on the lower part of the left eye and she did not flinch when a hat was waved before her eyes, also she lost her way in the bush trying to find the water hole.

Mrs Ferguson says: 'She is a very nervous horse, will not let anyone touch her and always flinches when saddled. She has a mean streak in her, probably due to former maltreatment, and will bite and kick other mares. I gave her Mimulus, Honeysuckle, Holly, Impatiens and Crab Apple. Mimulus for her nervousness; Honeysuckle for the memory of former maltreatment; Holly for jealousy and suspicion; Impatiens for her quick temper and Crab Apple to cleanse. Treatment began on 15 October.'

On 19 October Goldie's left eye had already cleared up. They waved a hat in front of her eyes and she flinched and, ridden up a narrow trail on the sand mountain, she did not have to be guided through the bush. No return of condition to date.

The Bach Centre Newsletter, March 1953

MR DARCY

When my wife and I purchased Mr Darcy, a beautiful grey, he was lame. We bought him to prevent him from being de-nerved (cutting off all feeling to his front foot). After this purchase we were at a loss as to what to do next, until my wife read an article in *Horse & Rider* magazine which described some help that a registered Bach practitioner, Stefanja Gardener, had given to two horses with emotional difficulties.

I called Stefanja for a chat. After our talk I was in a bit of a muddle – as an engineer I usually deal with facts whereas the remedies deal in emotions and feelings. But what was said seemed to tie in with what I could see with my new horse. He was head-shy, despondent, unresponsive, unhappy and lame. All in all a fairly pathetic creature. We decided to give him Gentian and Rescue Remedy and we were told to be patient, to wait, and to give him time.

We did – and Mr Darcy is a new horse. We were warned that progress would be slow, but that there was a character in there that was worth waiting for. I think we have seen some of it now and Mr Darcy is a very special horse. He has come on so well in the past three months that we have started looking at his physical side as well. He was examined by a chiropractor who put his pelvis back in place, his teeth have been done (they were in a frightful condition), he has special support shoes (egg-bars) – but most of all, he is now Mr Darcy. When the dentist was rasping he stood still because he knew that it would benefit him. He no longer balks at everything – he is not head-shy, he doesn't nod. He's not perfect, but he's as near to it as any of us are.

The other day Oscar, the horse in the next stable to Darcy, broke the fence and escaped. Darcy went with him. They spent a good hour galloping through corn fields and other places they weren't meant to be, until they were caught and put back into their stables. I went up to see them and was afraid that Darcy had hurt himself, but all I saw were two very hot, very sweaty but very happy partners-in-crime. I knew then that even if he never came sound at least he could make friends with other horses.

We both feel so grateful for Stefanja's gentle guidance and for our introduction to the Bach Flower Remedies. Without them I think we would still be floundering, and Darcy would still be suffering.

Mark & Geraldine Smith

CHAPTER 6:

On the Farm and in the Wild

Farm animals

'What is this life if, full of care,
We have no time to stand and stare.
No time to stand beneath the boughs
And stare as long as sheep or cows...'
Leisure, W.H. Davies

Life on the farm as depicted by children's story tellers is easy and pleasant, the nearest thing to heaven on earth. We can all picture it: the farmer leaning against the gate to the field, taking in the tranquillity of the setting, and contentedly watching his sheep grazing the lush grass; the farmer's wife happily making cakes in the warm kitchen, using freshly milled flour and home-produced butter; animals that are always healthy and happy and hardly need looking after – stories about farms where nothing ever goes wrong...

The reality is rather different. Whether running a large farm or simply keeping a few chickens and goats, working with farm animals is a balancing act between satisfaction in one area and responsibility and sacrifice in another. Despite the sense of freedom that working in the open air can bring, working with livestock can be as hectic and as worrying as any other job. Things do go wrong and often on a regular basis.

For both farmer and farm animal the remedies can be of great benefit. Farmers are comparatively easy to treat – but for obvious reasons it can be more difficult to select remedies for the twenty-fourth sheep in a herd of 300 than it is for your much-loved and much-observed pet cat. Despite the difficulties, however, it is still better where possible not to generalise too much. It may be tempting to consider all cows to be of a Wild Rose or Clematis nature and all sheep to be Cerato, but try not to be so blinded by the animal's caricature that the subtleties of its individuality go unnoticed. Farmers with a real interest in their animals often do notice individual characteristics even in large flocks, so it is possible to select remedies for individual animals even when, at first sight, they appear to be just one of the herd.

Particular situations will suggest specific remedies: a grieving mother would benefit from Star of Bethlehem, for example, while Walnut would help a new born, disorientated lamb to adjust to the next stage in its life. And of course for emergencies, Rescue Remedy is certainly the most basic and widely used remedy of all. It can be given to sheep, cows, pigs and goats in the throes of a difficult labour, and to the same animals in a state of shock following the birth of their young. It is the obvious remedy for all falls, injuries, shock, grief, terror, panic and hysteria, from chickens panicking after the visit of a fox, to cows frightened by low flying aircraft. And once the crisis is over you can reflect, at more leisure, on the individual remedies that might be useful. When you get to this point, the rule is the same as with all other animals: you are trying to relate to the animal's feelings and understand things from its point of view, thereby selecting the remedy or remedies that you think best suits the current need.

As with cats and dogs and horses, it is useful to know a bit about the particular species that you are going to treat, and the way it tends to act and react. For example, goats like to be active and have a tendency to rush around, which can cause problems if they injure themselves. Pregnant mothers may injure themselves or their unborn kids by trying to get through narrow gates too quickly, so Impatiens may be helpful at such times.

And of course it is especially important to separate out fact from legend, because legends about animals are not always correct. We all know stories about goats eating anything they can get hold of, and showing particular partiality to clothes drying on washing lines. But in fact goats can be fussy eaters, and like all animals that get used to certain foods they sometimes resist attempts to change their diets. Lois Hetherington in *All About Goats* tells of a goat who lived in a baker's yard in London until being bombed out in the Second World War. It was used to a diet of pastry, bread and apple peel left over from making fruit pies, and when it was evacuated to the countryside it refused, like a spoilt child, to touch its greens.

Farm case studies

UNCLE ARCHIE'S COW

In 1993 I was in the process of completing a four-day course about Bach Flower Remedies. The four days were split into two weekends with 12 weeks between them. During this time we had to prepare two case studies and one of mine was about Uncle Archie's cow.

Stephen, my husband, came home one Saturday afternoon after helping his uncle on his farm. He was a bit despondent and told me that his elderly uncle was contemplating putting down a cow as the animal had been sick for about six weeks and was getting progressively weaker and sicker, despite a number of visits from the vet and different courses of treatment.

Due to its ill condition it was unable to stand and had developed pressure sores on its underbelly. One of the front legs was beginning to contract.

After hearing this sad tale I asked Stephen if he thought Archie would consider letting the animal take the remedies. He felt that he would be willing as he was a great believer in the 'old ways' of healing.

Without further ado I prepared a treatment bottle. I used four drops of Rescue Remedy because it was an emergency situation. My gut feeling also told me to add two drops of the Oak remedy as the animal had been so brave to have battled on for so long.

The cow was in the field along with the rest of the herd, for company and also to give maximum 'grip' should she try to stand. Twenty-four hours after the first dose she was shakily attempting to stand and she received some help for a while from Archie. After that, her progress was rapid. Within a week her contracted leg had straightened and the pressure sores had healed. She appeared fully recovered.

In Uncle Archie's words, 'it was a miracle' – this from a gentleman who was in his seventies and had farmed all his days. He had never seen an animal recover having been down so long.

Serena Sheppard

SHEEP AND GOATS

I would like to share a few of my success stories with you.

Needless to say, Rescue Remedy is helpful whenever an animal is upset, distressed, in a panic or frightened. I once had a young orphan lamb that was tossed up in the air and landed on its back from a great height. The poor thing was in complete shock and after I had helped it to its feet it just stood stiff and wide-eyed. After one dose of Rescue Remedy it visibly got itself back together again within a few minutes and darted off.

The same lamb (he always had bad luck) got sunstroke one day and I found it open-mouthed and panting away in its pen. I applied cold water to head and legs and gave it a couple of doses of Rescue Remedy at half-hourly intervals. Recovery was quick and complete.

In both instances I half filled a 30 ml dropper bottle with spring water and added four drops of Rescue Remedy. I pushed the dropper into the side of the mouth, holding the head up slightly, and squirted the medicine down the lamb's throat. The tricky thing is that you have to be very careful so the animal doesn't bite the glass of the dropper.

The reason for only half filling the 30 ml bottle with spring water and then squirting in dropper-fulls of remedy is because one is bound to spill some of the medicine. Trying to administer four drops out of the dropper bottle each time, as you would do with humans, just won't do. You need to squirt in quite a bit more to make sure they at least get their four drops.

I have also been very successful in using the remedies on my goats. My goats are non-producing pygmy-goats; occasionally they have upset tummies.

Goats that are ill are very miserable creatures indeed. They just stand in a corner with their backs hunched and their hair standing on end. Keeping them indoors, feeding them only a little bit of hay or letting them fast for a day, combined with doses of Willow (to cheer them up) and Crab Apple, has always worked. Next day, improvement or complete recovery is guaranteed. If it is a mild case, I just add each remedy to a bucket of water which I place in the goat's pen.

My biggest success was with a pygmy-goat kid of a few months old that had rhododendron poisoning. The animal was in a very bad way when I found it, looking miserable, moaning softly and covered in green vomit. The vet was called out but he couldn't do anything apart from alleviate its stomach cramps. The poison would have to leave the animal the natural way, but it was quite possible she would die.

I decided to treat her myself. I chose Willow (to cheer the goat up so it would want to get better), Rescue Remedy (as it was in great distress and as its whole system seemed to be in shock and upset) and Crab Apple (to help it feel cleansed of the poison). The first two doses were given half-hourly. This resulted in another bout of heavy vomiting, which shocked me at first, but gave me a feeling of triumph as soon as I realised that this meant the poison was coming out.

When I came back an hour after the second dose the goat looked brighter and more interested in the world around her. I administered another dose. An hour later I came back again and found the animal walking around in her pen and even nibbling some hay. I gave her another dose. Yet another hour later I came back and the kid looked completely normal and contended. This was a miracle as far as I am concerned. Only four doses had given this result. I gave the animal a fifth dose and before locking the goats up for the night, a sixth. And that was that.

Petra Hofman

BUFFALO IN INDIA

A buffalo had a prolapsed uterus after giving birth which was corrected by a local villager. Three hours afterwards, the animal could neither eat nor drink, and her limbs and ears were cold. There was profuse bleeding and she was unable to stand.

I gave three doses of Rescue Remedy at 15 minute intervals. After the second dose, the uterus had again prolapsed and was bleeding, but the animal began eating hay and drinking water. A weak solution of Crab Apple was made with which the uterus cleansed. The uterus was then manipulated into position with ease. A few doses of Star of Bethlehem and Hornbeam (to overcome shock and give strength) were given at intervals of three hours. The animal was normal within 24 hours.

Bach Centre Newsletter, March 1954

STILLBORN CALF

A cow had delivered a calf in the night. The calf was dead and there was no trace of the placenta. I put the animal on to Star of Bethlehem for the first day and Crab Apple thereafter. After this, the placenta came away and the animal recovered completely.

Bach Centre Newsletter, March 1954

CHICKENS

My daughter had six chickens; during the coldest part of winter she was in the bedroom tidying up when she glanced out of the window to see a fox in the chicken run. Running like a demon downstairs, she was not in time to stop the fox from killing four of the chickens and making off.

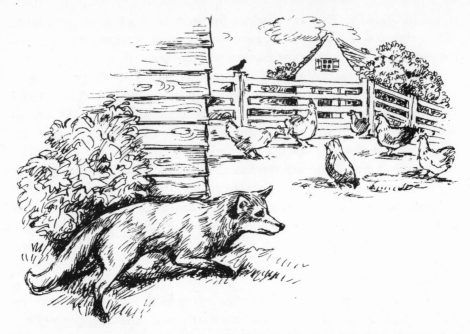

Very distressed and searching for the remaining two chickens, she heard a sound from behind a bush in the garden, and found the fifth chicken hiding there, badly hurt. The sixth chicken escaped unhurt.

My daughter took the injured chicken indoors and placed it in a box; its head was lolling to one side and there were puncture marks and blood over its body from the fox's attack. She trickled Rescue Remedy into its beak and bathed the wounds constantly with diluted Rescue Remedy. Within a very short space of time, the chicken began to respond.

But on the second day it was nothing short of a miracle. The chicken was already beginning to walk again, and even laid an egg, which must have been in its system when the attack took place. My daughter got some antibiotics the next day, as the wound to the body was obviously fairly serious, but the initial use of the Rescue Remedy undoubtedly saved its life. It is strutting around as happy as Larry now, none the worse for its escapade.

Kit Keetch

Wild animals

'I might just as well say, here and now, that in a very wide range of animals there is great individual variation in behaviour, and what I can only call 'character', within a species. By this I mean that if you had six toads, or six fox cubs, or six jackdaws, you would find among each half-dozen some that differed much in their ways and their temperaments from the others.'

Taming & Handling Animals, Maxwell Knight, 1959

Dr Bach's most fundamental rule when choosing remedies is to be mindful of the individuality of the person or animal being treated. We have seen many times in this book how this applies to animals like cats, dogs and horses. Maxwell Knight makes it clear that the same thing is true of wild animals.

The problem we face in trying to apply this insight is that we rarely have the time to get to know a wild animal. Even the farmer with his 300 sheep has a chance to get to know individuals in the flock, but when treating a wild animal typically we are in an emergency situation – and one that is not made easier by the fact that our patient's one overriding desire is to get away from us. Wild animals have an instinctive fear of predators and this means that they have an instinctive fear of man. If they are cornered and unable to get away their fear will probably emerge as aggression, which makes it not only difficult but potentially dangerous to try to get to know the animal.

What does this tell us about treating wild animals? In simple terms, this: if we do not have the leisure to identify type remedies, and if the patient is not co-operative, then we can still work on the mood remedy level alone. We may never know if the deer hit by a car is a Centaury or Vervain in its herd, but we do know that it is in an emergency situation and that it will be frightened – by our proximity if nothing else. Rescue Remedy is the main remedy to use, then, closely followed by fear remedies: Mimulus for the deer's fear of us; Cherry Plum if it is lashing out through fear and losing its self-control; Red Chestnut if it is aggressive in order to protect offspring. Needless to say, remedies like Vine for aggressive dominance are extremely unlikely to apply in such circumstances. Holly may have occasional uses, because it is the remedy among other things, for suspicion – but almost invariably a fear remedy is a more accurate choice.

The same general rules can be applied to any wild animal that you are likely to come across. And there are occasions in almost everyone's life when a wild animal, whether it be a baby hedgehog, a fox, a bird or a frog, is found injured or in distress and in need of some emergency help and comfort. Even if the injuries are so severe that the animal inevitably dies, the calming influence of the remedies, and of Rescue Remedy in particular, means that you can at least feel you have done something to help and so made its passing gentler and less traumatic.

And even when all hope seems to be gone there might still be hope. There have been many remarkable stories sent to us at the Bach Centre over the years, in which Rescue Remedy in particular has been crucial to the saving of an animal's life.

One personal memory is of a hedgehog that found its way into the garden pond one night. It was discovered in the morning, still in the water, but half drowned and exhausted by its repeated attempts to escape. Judging by the number of puncture marks in the pond liner it must have been in the pond most of the night.

Once free of the water it looked as if it was about to die. It was given Rescue Remedy diluted in some water and applied all around its mouth with the dropper and then it was gently placed in the shade under a big

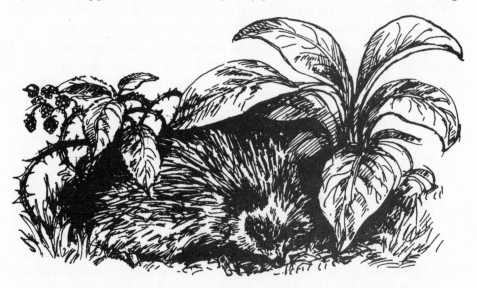

leaf. We expected it to die, but later in the day when we lifted the leaf the hedgehog had gone. It had recovered and made its escape as soon as it could.

Animals are extremely sensitive and have highly developed senses, particularly their hearing and smell. In addition, they seem to be highly sensitive to the negative emotions emanating from human beings. It has often been noticed how they tend to attack nervous people. It seems that human fear, even well disguised fear, makes animals afraid. They become either defensive and aggressive, or if they are themselves preda-tors, they may interpret a sense of nervousness as being evidence of prey, and will attack. Either way, the animal's aggression is fear driven, caused by our own fear of the animal concerned. But how do animals detect fear? Do they see it in the eyes? Can they smell it (possibly detect-ing adrenaline in the sweat)? Or do they tune in to some vague vibrational signal – something they can sense and we can't, just as we cannot hear some of the high pitched sounds which are audible only to dogs? The first suggestion would require a reasonable level of intelligence and intuition, so depending on your views, this may be a likely or very unlikely possibility. The second suggestion is probably the most accept-able explanation scientifically – although it does not explain how an animal or bird can detect fear at a distance. The third suggestion may require the most broad-minded acceptance of sixth sense phenomena, but nevertheless, is perhaps the most valid of all.

If we accept that animals tune in to fear, then it becomes especially important to consider our own feelings when faced with a potentially dangerous wild animal (all wild animals are potentially dangerous to some degree) that we want to help. We can start by acknowledging any reservations and nervousness that we feel. It's okay to feel like that, and okay, too, to use the remedies to remain in control of our fears. And if a situation feels like it may be beyond our ability to cope, we are also entitled (and obliged) to acknowledge this as well, and appeal for help before things get out of control.

Treating our moods and the moods of the suffering animal will help, but are we saying that it is never possible to go further? The answer is a resounding 'no'. It is always possible to go further if you are committed enough to what you want to do. Konrad Lorenz, famous for his work with greylag geese, was so experienced in his observation of posture and body language that he could tell how an individual goose felt just by looking at it. It is this type of non-verbal communication, which we looked at earlier in relation to the behaviour of more domesticated animals, that we can use to understand wild animals better and so find the remedies which most suit each individual animal's personality.

There is one situation where it *is* possible for people to get to know wild animals better as individuals and that, of course, is when they are in captivity. The problem here is that no matter how natural their cages are made to seem, they are still cages. They cannot ever replace the natural wild landscape or wilderness that their in habitants would naturally enjoy. Polar bears, tigers and other animals that pace back and forth relentlessly in their compound are bored and frustrated and, in a very real sense, are suffering from mental illnesses. In these circumstances the type remedy of the individual animal will in all likelihood be hidden beneath several layers of accumulated emotional stress. The answer to this is to treat one layer at a time, so begin by selecting remedies for the emotions you can see.

Similar repetitive behaviour is sometimes seen in caged birds, which can become almost manic as they squawk and peck repeatedly, clutching at one side of the cage, hurrying back along the perch and then clutching the other side, their eyes darting fervently from side to side. Behaviour such as this would indicate Cherry Plum for loss of control, and Impatiens for the hurried reaction – the urgent movements and the need to be free as quickly as possible. Rock Rose may also play an important part – terror and panic can easily escalate and become the cause of maniacal behaviour. This is why Rescue Remedy is so useful as it contains all three remedies: Cherry Plum, Rock Rose and Impatiens. In addition to these, Vervain should be considered as it is for the frustrated tension which is easily generated by an unfair and cruel situation. No bird that is not entirely tame and habituated to humans should have its freedom, natural curiosity and sense of enthusiastic energy so cruelly contained. The real remedy for any caged wild bird is to open the cage.

Wild animal case studies

A BLIND GULL
A lady who has a wild bird sanctuary in Saltash tells us of one of her gulls who had been poorly for many months and then developed a cataract:

'He became blind in one eye. For three days I gave him Mimulus for his fear as he kept dashing into things on his blind side, Hornbeam for he was fast losing strength, and Gorse for the hopelessness he must feel. You will be pleased to know that when I went to feed him this morning his blind eye was clear and he is able to see out of the eye. He was looking much happier.'

The Bach Centre Newsletter, March 1974

AN INJURED DEER

I am involved in deer management on a large estate in England and my phone is one of the first to ring when a deer has been knocked down on the estate roads. Normally when I arrive at the scene the poor beast has either died or the injuries are so bad that I have to put it down to save its suffering.

Two weeks ago, however, I was called out to find a three-year-old roebuck by the side of the road. It had some bad gashes on its back and rear and was in severe distress, although no bones seemed to be broken.

On this occasion I decided to take it home to see if I could do anything with it. I put it in a stable normally used by our Shetland pony and, having a bottle of Rescue Remedy handy, I managed to squeeze some drops into his mouth. I then left him to settle down for an hour or so.

When I looked in again he seemed a lot calmer, and I was able to take a closer look at his wounds. I bathed them and then applied some Rescue Cream.

What to give him in the way of nourishment would ultimately be a problem, as in the wild the roebuck's diet is enormously varied, with young shoots, herbs, flowers etc. For its first night, however, I thought it best to stick to the Rescue Remedy. The second time around there was

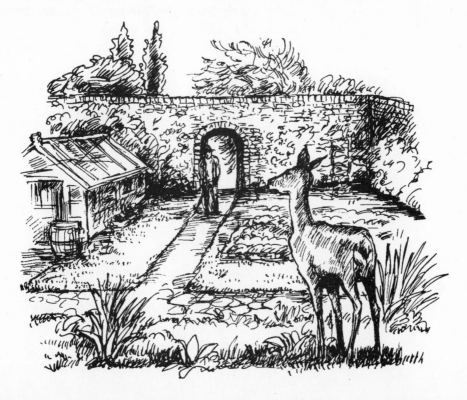

a definite licking of his lips after the first few drops.

I was very encouraged that he survived the first night and was convinced that the Rescue Remedy had calmed him down enough for me to tend to his wounds. I kept this up for two more days, slowly supplementing the Rescue with a bit of greenery. I had the vet look him over on the fourth day as one of his wounds needed some professional attention. Our vet practises homoeopathy and fully agreed with the use of Rescue. All the time the vet, her assistant and myself were poking around the buck's hind quarters he remained amazingly calm.

After the fifth day I decided to put him out into the walled back garden – perilously close to the vegetable patch – but he behaved himself, seeming content to eat the weeds and not my wife's plants.

By the eighth day he was becoming much stronger and less approachable, behaving more and more like the wild buck he was. His wounds were healing and there appeared to be no internal damage as his normal body functions seemed to be working okay.

So, two weeks to the day, I managed to corner and catch him and a friend and I took him to the woods and released him. There is no doubt in my mind that if it were not for the Rescue Remedy, calming and nourishing him in the first few days, he would not have survived.

Bach Centre Newsletter, December 1992

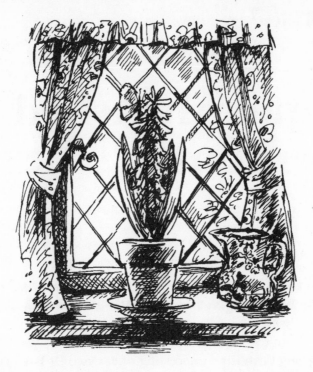

THE PREMATURE BUTTERFLY

In the middle of March while the weather was still very cold, we discovered a small copper butterfly obviously just free from her chrysalis. We took her indoors and for a whole week she slept on a vase of flowers.

Several times each day I sat her on a drop of Rescue Remedy on my finger, thinking that perhaps the vibrations might help to revive her. At last she unfurled her proboscis and took a long draught from the drop.

The result was immediate and almost startling. From being almost lifeless, she fluttered strongly about the room, but as the weather was still cold we kept her indoors for two more days, feeding her on fresh hyacinths and Rescue Remedy. At the end of that time, one sunny morning, we opened the window and watched her fly on strong wings to freedom.

The Bach Centre Newsletter, June 1951

CHAPTER 7:

Frequently Asked Questions

I work in a kennels helping bitches to whelp and as well as using the remedies to help my 'patients' I sometimes take Red Chestnut and Rescue Remedy myself.

Your point about treating yourself with Red Chestnut when one of your bitches is giving birth is an interesting one. Once Dr Bach cut his hand quite badly. When his helpers saw it obviously they were concerned, and he said then that their concern was like an extra burden for him to carry: the Red Chestnut helps to remove the burden of our worries from people (and animals) who are going through difficult or dangerous experiences.

My cat is scared of loud noises like fireworks, thunderstorms and even screaming children. When she is scared she shakes and runs around looking for somewhere to hide.

Mimulus would be helpful – it's the remedy for fear with a known cause. You might also try Rock Rose or Rescue Remedy, which will help to deal with the panicky feelings at particularly bad moments.

We have three great danes, all the same age and all female. One, Petra, is inclined to be overaggressive towards the others if she is excited for any reason (like when people come to visit). She especially dislikes any fuss being made of the other dogs.

Vine is the obvious remedy to give, as the problem certainly seems related to dominance. You might also find that if you make a point of making more of a fuss of Petra then the problem will ease.

We are nursing a hedgehog that is dying of cancer. It only has three or four weeks to live and we want to keep him comfortable. Is there anything that will help relieve his pain?

The Bach Flower Remedies do not treat physical symptoms directly, so a qualified vet should be consulted about pain relief and any other treatment that might be helpful. What the remedies can do is to help the animal to deal more effectively with how he is feeling and so help ease the transition for him. I would suggest Rescue Remedy, which contains remedies for terror and agitation and shock, plus Walnut to help him adjust to the great changes he is going through.

I imagine you are hurting too at the moment – you might find the remedies helpful yourself.

My cat has chronic renal failure. Our homoeopathic vet suggested using Rescue Remedy before his other treatments and it does seem to help him stay calm while we give him his fluids. Would any other remedies help his upset stomach? He is sick a lot, although the vet says there is nothing physically wrong....

The one that comes to mind is Crab Apple, which is the cleansing remedy and is good for feelings of sickness and contamination. It might also be possible to try to pinpoint other remedies for him by thinking about his personality generally – i.e. is he lazy, active, curious, friendly, shy etc.

...He is a fifteen year old tom. He is inquisitive and demanding, and likes people and animals and being held and petted – sometimes he is deliberately naughty just so as to be picked up. He has nightly cuddle sessions with the kids and gets really moody if they are away and he misses out. He loves running around the house with our two other cats as well, but is less interested in activity when they aren't around. Since the CRF treatment began, he has been very tired and doesn't run around as much as he used to.

From what you say I would guess that Chicory would be his type remedy – this is indicated by his affectionate and demanding nature, and by the way he loves having his 'family' around and gets depressed when he misses out on affection. I definitely think Olive would help him too – this is the remedy for tiredness caused by some effort – in this case the illness he has and his old age.

What remedies can I give to stop my dog from getting heartworm?
There aren't any remedies for specific illnesses, let alone for specific parasites. Instead the remedies are always selected for the personality and emotional state of the individual animal.

I have a ten year old rottweiler called Gerald. He has a diseased liver that is being treated by a homoeopathic vet. I have to travel on business a couple of times a year and when I go he gets really down, so the vet suggested giving him Rescue Remedy. I tried this, but it seemed to make Gerald depressed and lethargic.
The remedies don't give animals emotions that aren't already there, so there are two possible explanations. One is that Gerald was repressing these depressed feelings and they are being stirred up and released by the Rescue. If this is the case we would continue with the Rescue and, in addition, give other remedies to deal with the emotions released – exorcising them is part of the cure. Remedies that might be useful would include Gorse (feelings of hopelessness), Hornbeam (lack of energy at the thought of getting on with everyday activities) and Willow (self-pity). Walnut, Honeysuckle or Chicory might be useful when you have to go away on a trip.

The other possibility (especially in view of his liver problems) is that Gerald might be reacting to the brandy used to dilute the remedies. It would be a good idea to mention this possibility to the vet.

I gave Chestnut Bud to one of my horses to help with training, but it didn't make any difference. I've used Mimulus with the same animal and found it a great help, especially at show time. Any thoughts?
Chestnut Bud is good for when animals do not seem to notice patterns in their lives, or fail to learn from repeated experiences, but there might be a need for other remedies if a different kind of attitude is at the root of the problem. For example, a very strong-willed, dominant animal that thinks it knows better than you might need Vine, while a more apathetic character who simply isn't very interested in training could use Wild Rose. Does this suggest anything?

My dog is very clingy and dependent and cries if I go anywhere near the door. She also seems to be bursting with excess energy and gets very excited. I have given her Vervain for this and Chicory for the possessiveness. Is it worth adding Rescue Remedy as well?

Vervain and Chicory seem like good choices, and adding the Rescue Remedy should help to keep her calm generally. You might also think about Heather (needy, wrapped up in her own problems, desperate for any company – Chicory would be for a more choosy desperation for the family's company) and Mimulus (fear of a known thing, in this case your going away).

My three-year-old female pointer comes from a rescue home. At first she was very unsure of herself, but now, as her confidence grows, so does her aggressiveness. She is starting to become more dominant as well. My local behaviour counsellor suggested using the remedies, but I'm not sure which ones to try.

From what you have said it sounds like a Larch state (lack of confidence) is giving way to a more dominant form of behaviour that may be her underlying character. Remedies you might consider include Vine (she wants to get her own way and will be aggressive if that is the easiest way of getting it) and Chicory (she wants to be the centre of the family's attention and wants to be involved as leader in everything). You might also consider Rescue Remedy or Star of Bethlehem (often useful with rescue animals as they have been through traumatic times) and Walnut, which is the remedy to help her adjust to her new circumstances.

Our dog has suddenly developed a problem with licking – she won't stop licking at her feet, and she has turned her attention to the furniture as well, gnawing and licking at cushions and pillows. It's almost impossible to get her to stop.

Crab Apple is the remedy for this sort of obsessive behaviour. If you haven't already done so, you should consult a vet as well, as there may be other causes for this change in behaviour and that possibility needs to be investigated.

I have chosen six remedies that I think my rabbit needs to overcome a fear problem. Is it safe to mix that many together, and are there any combinations that I should avoid?

It's okay to mix up to seven together at a time, and there are no contra-indications within the system or with other medicines – any remedies from the 38 can be mixed together.

I work with a rescue home that rehouses unwanted dogs. We use Rescue Remedy to help ease the transition into a new family. Are there any other remedies that could help? And will we need the whole set?

The obvious remedy that you might find useful is Walnut, which is good for helping animals adapt to new surroundings and the different expectations put on them when they move home. And Star of Bethlehem will help animals suffering the effects of past traumas. Otherwise, though, you are right – in-depth use of the remedies for lots of different animals will inevitably mean that you will need to get the full set.

My cat Mopsie has skin cancer. I know the remedies don't treat this directly, but I want to help her feel more comfortable. She suffers terribly from itchy scabs on her skin – even before her illness she was quite withdrawn, and now it is worse. Do you have any suggestions?

Rescue Remedy is good for suffering animals, as it contains remedies to deal with feelings of agitation, fear, shock and distress. You might also try Crab Apple, which is the cleansing remedy. As you describe Mopsie as 'withdrawn' you might also consider whether any of the following are appropriate: Mimulus (for shy, timid creatures); Water Violet (for self-possessed, reserved animals who prefer their own company); Centaury (for gentle creatures who tend to be bossed around and do as they are told).

I am going to use Rescue Remedy on one of my cats on the advice of a friend, who also suggested Aspen. The cat has become very introverted lately following a move to a new town and another cat joining the family.

Aspen is for a vague foreboding, or fears that have no specific cause. It sounds like your cat has good reasons for his nervousness, so Aspen may not be appropriate. Rescue Remedy is a good choice, and you might also think about Walnut (for help adjusting to changed circumstances) and Mimulus (for fear of something you can name – perhaps the new cat).

A friend of mine rescued a pigeon that had been shot at with an air gun. The pigeon is on the mend but not able to fly, so my friend is having to feed and take care of it. However, the bird is still very timid and refuses to be tamed, and tries to get away and hide when anyone goes near.

There are three remedies you could consider: Mimulus for the fear of humans; Walnut to help adjust to the massive changes in its life; and Rescue Remedy to calm the bird down generally.

I have two dogs that both need remedies. What is the easiest way to give the remedies to them?

Normally the simplest way to give remedies is to put two drops of each individual remedy (four drops of Rescue Remedy) into the water bowl, and add more drops every time the bowl is refilled.

As you are treating two dogs and presumably are selecting different remedies for each, you could instead make up a treatment bottle for each animal by putting two drops of each individual remedy (four drops of Rescue Remedy) into an empty 30 ml dropper bottle (get these from the place you bought the remedies) topped up with still mineral water. From this bottle, give the dogs four drops four times a day – either dropped into their mouths, or on a small biscuit or some other treat.

Our dog, Buster, suffers from seizures and he gets restless for a few days before each attack. We use Rescue Remedy to help keep him calm – a few drops and he can get some sleep and stop pacing around for a time. This hasn't proved a long-term solution, however, and the seizures themselves are just as frequent and just as bad.

Rescue Remedy is designed for emergency use, which is why it isn't curing the problem, but is helping manage it. You might think about making up a personal mix of the remedies for Buster, selected according to what his personality is like and any particular emotions that he often shows (fear, excitement, dominance and so on).

I want to use the remedies on my goats – how much should I give them? The goats weigh anything from 110 up to 150 pounds.

The weight doesn't make any difference. You can make up an individual treatment bottle by putting two drops of each selected remedy (four of Rescue) into a 30 ml dropper bottle topped this up with still mineral water. From this bottle, give four drops, four times a day – either straight into the mouth or on a small edible treat.

If all the goats are having the same remedies you could, instead, add four to five drops of each selected remedy (10 of Rescue) into the water bucket or feed, and add further doses when the bucket or trough is refilled.

I have three mice that all share the same water bottle, but I only want to treat one of them. If I put the remedies in the bottle will they harm the mice that don't need the remedies?

There's no problem with the mice sharing the same bottle. If the other two don't need the remedies they will not experience any effects at all.

I've been giving remedies to our new dog, who we got from a dogs' home. His original owners abandoned him and now he howls the house down whenever we leave him in the house alone. At first, when I gave him Chicory and Star of Bethlehem, there was some improvement. Then I added Beech, Honeysuckle, Mimulus, Larch, Crab Apple and Wild Oat to the mix as well because I felt that there was more stuff in there that needed sorting out. Since then he seems to be going backwards.

Two suggestions – first, try giving fewer remedies, because at eight you are up around the limit and are probably giving a few that are not necessary. This will weaken the effect of the remedies that are necessary. Second – if Chicory and Star of Bethlehem alone were having a good effect it might be worth going back to them for a time, and only start assessing again when there is no further improvement from this mix.

My holistic vet has suggested I buy Rock Rose, Mimulus, Star of Bethlehem, Honeysuckle and Oak and give these to my Lipizzaner gelding. How do I go about giving them to him – mixed together or separately? How often do I give them? And can I put them in his feed or water? (He doesn't drink very much when in the stables, and soon he will be out in a field all day.)

There are two methods you could use. One is easier and the other is cheaper.

The cheaper method is to get hold of an empty 30 ml dropper bottle. Put two drops of each selected remedy in the bottle and top up with still mineral water. From this you need to give your horse four drops, four times a day – the easiest way to do this would be to put them on a sugar lump or some other treat that he will definitely eat.

The easier method uses a lot more remedy, since you can't be sure of the quantity of remedy he will be getting. This involves putting five drops of each remedy into his drinking bucket each time you refill it. Alternatively you could put the same mix into his food. This should ensure he gets the minimum dose even if he only takes a couple of swallows from time to time.

Our cat Bobo is a three-year-old, neutered male. He was never a problem until my daughter left her cat, who is an unneutered male, with us while she went away for a weekend. At once Bobo began spraying the carpet, beds, chairs and sofas, and he hasn't stopped since, even though the visiting cat went home weeks ago. Our vet has put him on an anti-anxiety drug called Elavil, which is controlling the problem, but if you take him off the drug he goes back to spraying again.

It sounds like he is trying to reassert himself and mark out his space. (I wonder if there might be traces of the rival cat's smells about the house that he is trying to cover over?) The obvious remedies to try are Rescue Remedy, Mimulus and Vine. Star of Bethlehem would help him over any unresolved shock created by this or by the visitor cat. Walnut or Honeysuckle might help him to move on as well – and since he is still repeating a behaviour that was necessary in the past, when the other cat was there, but is no longer appropriate, I would tend to go for Honeysuckle. He also seems to lack self-confidence, so Larch might be a good idea as well.

I recently bought some Rescue Remedy on the recommendation of a friend. It is for my Bichon Frise dog. She likes going to our dog training group and gets very excited and a bit hyper. This is a problem because I want to enter her for kennel club obedience trials, and I'm worried she'll get worked up and lose control. Is Rescue Remedy the right choice for this situation? If it is, will it make her drowsy, because I need her alert if she is going to perform well?

Yes, it will help calm her down, and it won't make her tired or have any negative effects. You might also consider using Vervain, which is specifically for overenthusiasm.

I have a cob who every year gets bitten by midges and suffers an allergic reaction – the condition is called sweet itch. Usually he is a dependable, sturdy horse, but when the sweet itch comes he becomes distressed and hard to handle. We use a product called KillItch, and lavender, and these seem to help – can the Bach Flower Remedies help as well?

You might think about the following: Crab Apple to help cleanse him of the itching; Cherry Plum to help him keep his self-control; Impatiens for the agitation he feels. I wondered also about Elm, as he sounds like he copes with things well normally but finds this particular problem more than he can handle. You could try giving these remedies to him, but of course they won't stop the midges from biting!

I keep a few goats and we had a nasty incident a while ago when one of them was killed by a dog. I have been giving the rest of them Rescue Remedy very frequently for a few weeks now, but I'm concerned about giving them too much.

You can't overdose on the remedies and they aren't habit forming or dangerous in any way, so there is no danger of giving them too much. Simply give them as frequently as needed until the problem has gone.

My dog trainer suggested I use Rescue Remedy for our new puppy who is not yet six months old. Like most young dogs, he is a bit hyperactive and loses his temper quite a bit. We are hoping the Rescue will help us through the next few months until he grows up a bit.

Rescue Remedy is often used with animals to help calm them down, especially at times of stress. You might also try Cherry Plum to help him control his temper, and Vervain for his excitability. You can give both of these at the same time as the Rescue Remedy – they are absolutely safe, even for very young animals.

Small animals and birds have a much higher rate of metabolism than people, so is it necessary to increase the dosage to compensate for this?

No. You can make up a treatment bottle in the normal way or you can put two drops into the water bowl or bottle (four drops of Rescue Remedy), which is the equivalent to a human having two drops in a glass of water.

How quickly do the remedies work if you give them for feelings related to a specific situation?

For short-term emotions the results can be very quick – however, if the response to the situation is an ongoing one, for example, if your dog always becomes fearful in company and has done so for some time, then this would count as a long-term problem and it may take several weeks before you begin to see an improvement.

Our cat is spraying. Any ideas?

Cats can spray for all kinds of reasons – you simply need to look at the reason and then treat that. In many cases it is anxiety-based, so Mimulus/Rescue Remedy can be considered. If there has been a change in the cat's life that triggered an increase in spraying, that can be a clue to the cause.

CHAPTER 8:

Going on from Here

Learning more about the remedies

Dr Bach's dream for his system was that everyone should be able to use it. Accordingly, there are a number of ways that you can learn more about his remedies and about how to use them, not only on animals, but also on yourself, your friends and your family.

BOOKS
There are hundreds of books available on the remedies and, as with any other subject, the quality and accuracy of the information available varies. One way to choose books is to look for the 'Bach Centre Recommended' logo on the front cover.

All the following books are published by Vermilion:

- *Bach Flower Remedies Step by Step* by Judy Ramsell Howard – the simplest general introduction to the remedies, with indications for all 38 and all the basic information you need to select and use them.
- *The Bach Remedies Workbook* by Stefan Ball – a complete course in learning to use the remedies, with lots of games, quizzes and activities to help you learn your way around the system.
- *Bach Flower Remedies for Women* by Judy Ramsell Howard – a chronological survey of a woman's life with suggestions for using the remedies at each stage.
- *The Illustrated Handbook of the Bach Flower Remedies* by Philip M. Chancellor – in-depth descriptions of Remedies with colour Bach Flower illustrations.

- *The Essential Writings of Dr Edward Bach* by Dr Edward Bach with a preface by Judy Ramsell Howard – Dr Bach provides insight into the 38 remedies using his own words.
- *Dictionary of the Bach Flower Remedies* by T. W. Hyne Jones – lists the positive and negative aspects of the 38 remedies to help you find the remedy you need.

CASSETTES
- *Getting to Know the Bach Flower Remedies is a useful aide memoire* published by the Bach Centre: side one contains descriptions of all 38 remedies, while side two provides exercises for practice – and gives you the answers as well.

VIDEOS
- *Bach Flower Remedies: A Further Understanding* is a video produced by the Bach Centre featuring interviews with the trustees who explain in a simple and straightforward way how the remedies should be used.
- *The Light That Never Goes Out* is another Bach Centre video, this time telling the story of Dr Bach's live and work and how both found a permanent home at Mount Vernon.

COURSES
If you are someone who learns best in the company of other people then there are a number of different courses that you might want to take.
- *Independent courses* are run all round the world. The advantage is that they are local and usually inexpensive; the disadvantage is that, like the books, the quality and accuracy of teaching varies. If possible look for a course run by a qualified registered practitioner – the Bach Centre may know of one near you.
- *Official Courses – Level 1.* The Dr Edward Bach Foundation and A. Nelson & Co., who distribute the remedies around the world, have put together a three-stage series of courses designed to teach all the basics of using this therapy. The Level 1 Course is aimed at complete beginners, but even people who know the remedies quite well can benefit from a course that gives a clear view of all 38 remedies as well as the chance to ask acknowledged experts in the use of the remedies those questions that you can't find answers for in books. To apply, see the **useful addresses** section on page 153.
- *Official Courses – Level 2.* The Level 2 Course is for more advanced

users of the remedies. Among other things, it makes clear some of the subtle differences between pairs of remedies, and explores the concepts of type and mood remedies. To apply, see the **useful addresses** section on page 153.

- *Official Courses - Level 3.* The Level 3 Course is really aimed at people who want to work professionally with the remedies. As well as four days' training there is an exam to pass and a study period of up to six months during which students prepare essays and case studies of actual clients they are treating. After the course has been success fully completed, students are offered the chance to accept a Code of Practice and be included on the International Register of Practitioners maintained at Mount Vernon by the Dr Edward Bach Foundation. To apply, see the **useful addresses** section on page 153.
- *Correspondence Courses.* There are many correspondence courses being offered in the remedies. The authors of this book have not examined all of them, but the ones we have seen are overpriced and inaccurate. If you are thinking about investing in a correspondence course, our advice is to be careful before parting with money, and to be especially wary of correspondence courses that offer diplomas or certificates or purport to equip you for work as a professional practitioner. The Dr Edward Bach Foundation is considering the introduction of a correspondence course equivalent to the official Level 1 Course (see above), but at the time of writing these plans are at a very early stage.
- *Special Courses.* The Dr Edward Bach Foundation runs a few courses every year specifically for people who want to use the remedies to help animals. These are designed for registered practitioners, but are open to members of the public as well. Places are limited, and applicants are expected to know all 38 remedies and to have attained a standard equivalent to having followed the official Level 2 Course. Contact the Bach Centre for more details.

MAKING THE REMEDIES PART OF YOUR LIFE

Dr Bach wanted people to think of and use the remedies in an entirely natural way, just as they use water, air and food. It follows that learning to use the remedies properly means more than simply memorising a list of indications and dosage instructions. It means finding ways to make the remedies part of your life.

The best and most obvious way to do this is to use them yourself. Read back through the remedy descriptions in Chapter 2 and make a note of any that ring a particular chord with you. You might start by thinking that you need all 38, and this is true in a way since all the states are normal states to be in, and all of us can suffer from them at different stages of our lives. But try to narrow things down to one or two remedies that seem to describe you as a person, rather than the transient moods you are going through. The one or two remedies you end up with could be your type remedies.

Next think about how you feel right now. Perhaps you are entirely happy and content and in a very positive state of mind. If so, you don't need to take any remedies. But if you feel tired, irritable or lonely, then you could take some time to try to pinpoint the remedies that will help you with this.

You might feel that you need to make yourself up a treatment bottle, or you might feel that you only need to treat a passing mood or two. Either way, don't make this process of selecting remedies a one-off event, but instead try to think about the remedies you need on a day-by-day basis. And having considered the remedies, if there are some that you need, then go ahead and take them.

You will almost certainly find that as you consider your own need for remedies so you will begin to be more aware of the states of minds and personality types of the people around you as well. Thinking about what remedies other people might need is an excellent way of learning the indications and beginning to 'think Bach'. And you can extend the principle to fictional characters too: from Shakespearian tragedy and Greek myth to the latest soap opera, any character with any life at all will be reflected in the 38 remedies of Dr Bach, and matching character to remedy is another good way of learning your way around the system.

Now this approach might sound to some overintense or even fanatical, but it is not meant to be. If you think about it we are used to applying categories to everything, including living beings. We use quite technical words like extrovert, introvert, psychotic and neurotic to describe characters and behaviour, because those words have passed into the common language and are readily understood by most people. This is all you are doing when you start to think about personality and soul using the names of the remedies as your labels. But instead of just being labels to stick on things the remedies are wonderfully simple tools that allow us to heal and to turn negative, harmful emotions into positive ones. Once you have leanrt to think Bach then the remedies really will be part of your life and Dr Bach's wish, as passed down to us by Nora Weeks in her biography, will have been fulfilled:

'I want to make it as simple as this: I am hungry, I will go and pull a lettuce from the garden for my tea; I am frightened and ill, I will take a dose of Mimuius.'

Learning more about animals

BOOKS
This is an informal bibliography of the books consulted in the course of researching and writing this book. They are listed in alphabetical order by author.

- Fogle, Bruce, *The Cat's Mind,* Pelham Books, London, 1991
- Fogle, Bruce, *The Dog's Mind,* Pelham Books, London, 1990
- Hetherington, Lois, *et al. All About Goats,* Farming Press, Ipswich, third revised edition 1992
- Knight, Maxwell, *Taming and Handling Animals,* G. Bell & Sons, London, 1959
- Lorenz, Konrad, *On Aggression,* Methuen & Co, London, 1966
- Masson, Jeffrey and McCarthy, Susan, *When Elephants Weep,* Vintage, London, 1996
- McHattie, Grace, *That's Cats!,* David & Charles, Newton Abbot, 1991
- Morris, Desmond, *Catwatching,* Ebury Press, London, 1994
- Morris, Desmond, *Illustrated Horsewatching,* Ebury Press, London 1997
- Tabor, Roger, *Understanding Cats,* David & Charles, Newton Abbot, 1995
- Tellington-Jones, Linda and Taylor, Sybil, *Getting in Touch with Horses,* Kenilworth Press, Buckingham, 1995
- Villee, Claude, Walker, Warren, and Barnes, Robert, *General Zoology,* CBS College Publishing, Holt Saunders International, 1984

OBSERVATION AND PRACTICE
As with learning about the remedies, so with animals: reading is a good preparation but to really know the subject you have to live with it. Most people reading this book will have at least one animal in their family, and that is the best place to start. Notice what your animal does, and try to interpret its behaviour. Think about the behaviour in remedy terms, and use the remedies you select to help the animal achieve balance.

To some extent this involves reading your own emotions into the animal and assuming that it is feeling and reacting the way you would if you were in that situation. There is obviously a danger when doing this, which is that you will interpret things with no regard for the differences in social organisation and world view that exist between us and other animals, and between different species of other animals. Read back through this book, and especially the early chapters, to remind yourself of the usefulness and the potential problems of identifying your own emotions with those of the animals around you.

You can also get a lot of useful information from television: there are hundreds of top-quality programmes all year round on animals, where experts talk you through the why's and wherefores of animals' lives. You can gain real insight from these programmes, but beware the tendency to over-anthropomorphise that is shown by some presenters and film producers.

Finally, see if there are any local clubs or societies with a particular interest in the animals you are most passionate about. The library is a good place to start your research, or the local paper might be able to help. You might also contact your nearest college to see if they run courses on animal psychology or animal behaviour. These are all good ways to learn more, and to meet people with tales to tell. You might even be asked to help people to select remedies for their animals, which might be the start of a whole new way of life...

Useful addresses – Bach Flower Remedies

THE DR EDWARD BACH CENTRE

Mount Vernon is the small Victorian cottage that Dr Bach chose to be the centre of his work. Over the years, the team who work there and the place itself have come to be known as the Bach Centre. Their main role and responsibility is to make the mother tinctures for the Bach Flower Remedies, a task which has been handed on to them by direct succession from Dr Bach himself. The house and garden are open to visitors, and free help and advice on using the remedies is given by letter, phone and e-mail. Callers can also be referred to trained practitioners who are registered with the Dr Edward Bach Foundation (see below). The business arm of the Centre, The Bach Centre Mount Vernon Ltd., supports all its other activities and runs a shop at the Centre which stocks books, tapes, videos, postcards and many other items, most of which are also available by mail order.

Address: Mount Vernon, Bakers Lane, Sotwell, Wallingford, Oxon OX10 0PZ, England
Tel: 00 44 (0) 1491 834678
Fax: 00 44 (0) 1491 825022
E-mail: centre@bachcentre.com
WWW: http://www.bachcentre.com

THE DR EDWARD BACH FOUNDATION

The Dr Edward Bach Foundation was set up by the Bach Centre in the early 1990s. It is the educational arm of the Centre, and started training practitioners in 1991. By 1999 there were well over 500 on its register. Working with the Education Department at A. Nelson & Co. (see below), it has been active in setting up official training courses in many different parts of the world, from New Zealand and Japan to France and Holland.

Address: Mount Vernon, Bakers Lane, Sotwell, Oxon OX10 0PZ, England
Tel: 00 44 (0) 1491 834678
Fax: 00 44 (0) 1491 825022
E-mail: foundation@bachcentre.com

THE DR EDWARD BACH HEALING TRUST

This is the charitable wing of the Bach Centre and was set up to spread Dr Bach's system and message of self-help by gifts of money and remedies made to deserving causes and to individuals working with the remedies under difficult circumstances. As well as this work, the Trust owns the house and garden of Mount Vernon, so ensuring that it will continue as the centre of his work for all time, as Dr Bach intended.

Address: Mount Vernon, Bakers Lane, Sotwell, Oxon OX10 0PZ, England

Tel: 00 44 (0) 1491 834678

Fax: 00 44 (0) 1491 825022

E-mail: trust@bachcentre.com

A. NELSON & CO. LTD./BACH FLOWER REMEDIES LTD.

In 1991 the Bach Centre asked the homoeopathic company A. Nelson & Co. Ltd., with whom they had been closely acquainted since Dr Bach himself first supplied Nelsons Pharmacy with tinctures, to take over exclusive responsibility for bottling and worldwide distribution of the remedies prepared from its mother tinctures. Nelsons' expertise in this area has meant that the remedies are now available in many more countries than used to be the case, and their experience with licensing and legal matters has made the remedies much more secure against potential threats from future regulation of complementary medicine. As the worldwide distributors, Nelsons are the best people to contact for information about local availability of the remedies wherever in the world you live.

Nelsons have also contributed greatly to the education programme, setting up and administering the Bach International Education Programme in association with the Dr Edward Bach Foundation.

Address: Broadheath House, 83 Parkside, London SW19 5LP, England

Tel: 00 44 (0) 181 780 4200

Fax: 00 44 (0) 181 780 5871

Other useful addresses

- APACHE (The Association for the Promotion of Animal Complementary Health Education), Archers Wood Farm, Coppingford Road, Sawtry, Huntingdon, Cambridgeshire PE17 5XT, England. Tel: 07050 244196. E-mail: apache@avnet.co.uk. Web site: www.avnet.co.uk/~apache/

- Battersea Dogs Home, 4 Battersea Park Road, London SW8 4AA, England. Tel: 0171 622 3626. Web site: www.dogshome.org
- British Homoeopathic Veterinary Association, Chinham House, Stanford-in-the-Vale, Faringdon, Oxfordshire SN7 8NQ, England.
- PDSA (People's Dispensary for Sick Animals), White Chapel, Priorslee, Telford, Shropshire TF2 9PQ, England. Tel: 01952 290999.
- RSPCA (Royal Society for the Prevention of Cruelty to Animals), Causeway, Horsham, West Sussex RH12 1HG, England. Tel: 01403 264181.

Index

accidents *see* injuries
Adam: and animals 1
addresses, useful 153–5
administration of remedies *see*
    dosage
aggression: and fear
    in cats 53–4, 57–9
    in dogs 68–9
    in wild animals 133–4
    see also dominance aggression
Agrimony 7, 17, 47, 51
    case study (cat) 96
alcohol: in remedies 40, 102, 140
allergies
    in dogs 70–1
    in horses 122–3, 145
aloofness: remedy 36
Animal Behaviour 12
anthropomorphism 8–9, 10–11,
    152
    and body language 9, 60
anxiety/apprehension 17, 69
APACHE 154
apathy: remedy 37
Arcouet, Lucille 81
Aspen 7, 17–18, 69, 142

Bach, Edward ix, 4–6, 138
    on personality 11–12
    and physical type 65
    remedies: system 6–8
    on simplicity 13–14, 40–1,
        150, 151
    writings 147, 148
Bach (Dr Edward) Centre
    153
Bach Centre Mount Vernon
    Ltd. 153
Bach (Dr Edward) Foundation
    41, 43, 153
    Code of Practice 41, 43
    courses 149–50
Bach (Dr Edward) Healing Trust
    154
Bach International Education
    Programme 154
Ball, Stefan xi, 147, 148
barking: meaning 51–2
Barnes, Robert 152
bats: and echo location 9
Battersea Dogs Home 155
Becker, Patricia Reeve-De 97
Beech 18, 54

behaviour
  and breed 63–6
  and gender 62–3
  problems 105–7
    apparent 8–10
      in horses 119, 120–1
    in cats 8–9, 85–90, 106–7,
      139, 142
    in dogs 9, 64, 105–7, 138,
      140–6
    see also scent marking
  and species 8–10
behaviourism 2
bereavement 71, 104
birds 49, 61
  in captivity 134
  treatment 101–2, 132, 146
    examples 134, 142
bitterness: remedy 37–8
blindness 81, 123, 134
body language 48–9, 52–62,
    110–12, 113–14, 133
  and anthropomorphism 9, 60
books: on remedies 147–8
brandy: in remedies 40, 102, 140
breeds: and behaviour 63–6
British Homoeopathic Veterinary
    Association 155
Bruce, Ann 101
buffalo: treatment 129
Bullen, Victor xi
Burling, Joy E. 79
butterfly: case study 137

cancer 92–3, 139, 142
captivity, animals in 69, 133–4
carers/owners, treating 104–7,
    138
cassettes: on remedies 148
castration: effects 62

cats 9, 82–90
  aggression and fear 53–4, 57–9
  behaviour
    and breed 64–5
    and gender 62–3
    problems 8–9, 85–90, 106–7,
      139, 142
  case studies 90–101
  communication
    non-verbal 52–9, 61–2
    verbal 49–52
  dosage 39–41
  eating problems 89–90, 93,
    106
  and fear 58–9, 94–5, 98–9,
    100, 138
Centaury 18–19, 29
Cerato 19
Chancellor, Phillip 148
change
  coping with: remedy 35
  as stressor in cats 87–8, 90
cheerfulness: masking suffering
    17
Cherry Plum 7, 8, 19, 38, 69, 131
Chestnut Bud 20, 140
chickens: case study 129–30
Chicory 20–1, 25, 31, 100
chimpanzees 61
Cierniak, Britta 104
cleaning see grooming
cleansing remedy see Crab Apple
Clematis 22, 38
cocker spaniels 64
communication
  non-verbal see body language
  verbal 49–52
confidence, lack of 28
Courage, Vanessa 77
courses 149–50

cows: case studies 127, 129
Crab Apple 19, 22–3, 69, 142
  in Rescue Cream 38, 39
criticism of others 18

Davies, W.H. 125
Day, J.E. 104
daydreaming: remedy 22
deer: treatment 131, 135–6
defensiveness *see* fear
depression: remedies 23–4, 29,
  34
Descartes, René 2
despair: remedy 34
direction, lack of 36–7
discouragement 23–4
Dobermanns 64
dogs 9, 67–72, 105–6
  aggression and fear 68–9
  behaviour
    and gender 63
    problems 9, 64, 105–7, 138,
     140–6
  case studies 73–81
  communication
    non-verbal 59–61
    verbal 51–2
  dosage 39–41, 143
  training 78, 145
dominance: remedy 35
dominance aggression
  in cats 58, 82
  in dogs 69–70, 76–7, 138, 141
dosage 39–41
  by animal
    birds 102, 146
    cats 39–40
    dogs 39–40, 143, 144
    goats 128–9, 143, 146
    horses 40, 144

    lambs 128
    small animals 143–4, 146
  mixing remedies 39, 141, 144

ears: in body language 62
  of cats 53–4
  of dogs 59
  of horses 110–11
eating problems
  in cats 89–90, 93, 106
  in dogs 70–1
elephants 10
Elm 23
emergencies *see* injuries; Rescue
  Remedy
emotions
  in animals 10–11
  sensing of 105, 132–3
  in treatment 6–7, 16
envy: remedy 25–6
escapism, mental 22
exhaustion: remedy 30
eyes: of cats 54–6

farm animals 125–30
fatigue: remedies 26, 30
fear
  in animals:
    cats 57–9, 138
     case studies 94–5, 98–9,
     100
    dogs 60–1, 68–9, 74
     and owners 105
    horses 109, 111, 115, 118
     and riders 117
    smaller 101–2
    wild 131, 132–3
  types: and remedies 6–7, 69
    acute (terror) 32
    of everyday things 28–9

of insanity 19
  for others 12, 31
  vague 17–18
fish 61, 103–4
fits (seizures) 78, 143
flehming 9
foals 112–13
Fogle, Bruce 10, 57, 151
Fox and the Hound 67
foxes 132
frogs 132

Gardener, Stefanja 124
gender: and behaviour 62–3
Genesis, book of 1–2
Gentian 23–4
Glidden, Patrick 13
goats 65–6
  dosage 143, 146
  treatment 126–9
goldfish 103–4
Gorse 24
grooming, excessive 19, 69, 96,
  141
guilt: remedy 31
guinea pigs 104

Hahnemann, Samuel 5
hamsters: and fear 102
hatred: remedy 12, 25–6
Heather 24–5, 79, 87
hedgehogs 132, 139
Hetherington, Lois 126, 151
Hippocrates 13, 15
Hofman, Petra 129
holism: concept 15–16
Holly 8, 12, 25–6, 131
  care over use 26, 68, 69, 70
homoeopathy 5, 44
Honeysuckle 26

hopelessness: remedy 24
Hornbeam 26
horses
  allergies 122–3, 145
  body language 61, 110–12
  case histories 122–4
  character: and physique 65
  control 27–8
  dosage 40, 144
  as herd animals 9, 108–13,
    115–16, 120
  injuries/emergencies 118–20,
    122–3
  and riders 113–18
  riding as therapy 104
  showing/competing 121
  and stables/horse-boxes 120–1
  training 113, 117, 140
Howard, Judy xi, 147, 148

imbalance: remedy 33
impatience: remedy 27–8
Impatiens 27–8, 38
indecision: remedy 33
injuries/emergencies
  and farm animals 126–30
  and horses 118–20, 122–3
  and small animals 102–4
  and wild animals 131–2,
    135–6
  see also Rescue Remedy
injustice, sense of: remedy 34
insanity, fear of 19
intelligence: of animals 3
internet 44
intolerance: remedy 18
irritability: remedy 27–8

jealousy: remedy 25–6
Jones, Barbara 76

Kaplan, Lucy 94, 99
Keetch, Kit 130
kidney disease 96–7, 139
Knight, Maxwell 131, 151

Larch 28–9, 68
law: and remedies 41–3
lethargy 26
Lewis, Betty 74
Li, Shirley 93
licking *see* grooming
liver disease 78–9, 140
Lorenz, Konrad 12–13, 133, 151

machines, animals as 2–3, 15
Masson, Jeffrey 151
McCarthy, Susan 151
McHattie, Grace 151
medicine, Western 15–16
Merrifield, Charlotte 78
mewing: meaning 51
mice: and dosage 143–4
Midgley, Clare 76
Mimulus 6, 28–9, 31, 54, 68, 69,
    131
mind: and body 4
mistakes, inability to learn from
    20
Mitchell, Marion 78
Moelk, Mildred 49
monkeys: alarm calls 49
Morris, Desmond 51, 151–2
Mount Vernon 153, 154
Mourant, Jenny 96
Mustard 7, 29, 63

Nelson (A.) & Co. 153, 154
neonatal care 78
nettle allergy: case 122–3
neutering: effects 62–3

Newman, Chris 93
Nieder, Jeannette 74
Noah: and animals 1

Oak 29–30, 51
obesity: in cats 89, 106
Occam's razor 10
Olive 26, 30
overprotectiveness 12
owners/carers, treating 104–7,
    138

pair bonding: in horses 109–10
panic: remedy 32
Paracelsus 15
parasites 140
past, preoccupation with: remedy
    26
Pavlov, Ivan Petrovich 68
PDSA 155
perfectionism 18
personality 11–12
    and animals 12–13
    traits: and remedies 7–8
pessimism: remedy 24
Pine 31
possessiveness 20–1
    case study 99–100
posture: in body language
    of cats 57–9
    of dogs 59–61
    of horses 111–12
    of humans 113–14
Prestwich, Anne 95
pride: remedy 36
purring: meaning 50–1
Pythagorus 13

rabbits 9, 101, 102–3, 141
Raffels, Madeleine 98

Ramsell, John xi, 148
Red Chestnut 7, 12, 31–2, 69,
    107, 131, 138
  for female dogs 63, 78
referrals: from vets 42–3, 44–5,
    152
renal disease 96–7, 139
Rescue Cream 38–9
Rescue Remedy 38, 44, 118
  in dog training 78, 145
  in emergencies:
    liver disease 78–9, 140
    near strangulation 73–4
    neonatal care 78
    seizures 78, 143
  in treating
    cats 54, 142
    birds 134
    butterfly 137
    deer 131, 135–6
    farm animals 126, 127–9,
      130
    horses 28, 118, 122–3
    small animals 102–3
    wild animals 131–2
resentment: remedy 37–8
resignation: remedy 37
resilience 29–30
responsibility, being
  overwhelmed with 23
Richards, Lyn 78
riding, horse- 104, 113, 114–15,
    117–18
rigidity, mental 32–3
Rock Rose 6, 32, 38, 54, 69
Rock Water 7, 16, 32–3
Rogerson, Christina 95
Rottweilers 64, 140
RSPCA 155

Sade, Marquis de 2–3
Sampson, Elisa 100
Sanders, Judith 74, 100
scent marking 52
  in cats 87–8, 93–4, 145, 146
  in dogs 70, 71
Scleranthus 33
seizures 78, 143
selection: principles 46–9
self-absorption 24–5
self-confidence: lack 28
self-denial: remedy 32
self-distrust 19
self-doubt: remedy 19
selfishness: remedy 20–1
self-pity: remedy 37–8
self-reproach: remedy 31
separation anxiety 105–6
  case studies 76, 79
sheep 126, 127–8
Sheppard, Serena 127
shock: remedy 33–4
shyness: remedy 28–9
simplicity: of remedies 14, 40–1,
    150, 151
Skinner, B.F. 2
small animals 101–4
  dosage 143–4, 146
  see also birds
smell, sense of 9, 52, 105
Smith, Geraldine 124
Smith, Mark 124
songbirds see birds
souls: and animals 11–14
spaniels, cocker 64
spaying: of cats 62–3
species: and behaviour patterns
    8–10
specificity
  of illnesses 140

of situations 146
spongillosis: case study 80
spraying *see* scent marking
stallions 108–9
Star of Bethlehem 7, 33–4, 38
storms, fear of 74, 100, 138
strangulation, near: case study
   73–4
stress: and diagnosis 71, 90
submissiveness: in dogs 59–60, 70
suspicion: remedy 25–6
Sweet Chestnut 34

Tabor, Roger 152
tail: in body language
   of cats 56–7
   of horses 111
Taylor, Sybil 152
Tellington-Jones, Linda 65, 152
terminal care 75, 92
   of wild animals 131, 139
territorialism 71–2, 83
terror: remedy 32
timidity: remedy 28–9
tiredness: remedies 26, 30
training 105, 107
   of dogs 78, 145
   of horses 113, 117, 140
trauma
   case studies 81, 95
   as shock: remedy 33–4
   see also injuries; Rescue
      Remedy
type remedies 7–8

Uittenbogaard, Bianca 79, 98, 103
uncertainty: body language 61

urination *see* scent marking
US Army: therapy programme
   104

Vervain 28, 34
vets: and remedies 42–3, 44–5,
   152
videos: on remedies 148
Villee, Claude 152
Vine 8, 35, 54, 98
   use with dogs 69, 138
vocal utterances 48, 49–52
vomiting: case study 97–8

Walker, Warren 152
Walnut 35, 87, 114
Water Violet 7, 36, 47, 86, 87
weakness of will 18–19
weariness: remedies 26, 30
Weeks, Nora ix, xi, 36, 46, 47,
   90–2, 148
weight *see* eating problems
whining: in dogs 51
whiskers: use 54
White Chestnut 16, 36
wild animals 131–6
   body language 61, 133
   in captivity 69, 133–4
   terminal care 131, 139
   see also birds
Wild Oat 36–7
Wild Rose 26, 37
Willow 21, 37–8
worrying: remedy 36
Wumps ix, 36

York Retreat 104

ALSO AVAILABLE FROM VERMILION

☐ Bach Flower Remedies for Women	0091906547	£7.99
☐ The Essential Writings of Dr Edward Bach	0091906725	£4.99
☐ Illustrated Handbook of the Bach Flower Remedies	0091906482	£12.99
☐ The Bach Flower Remedies Step by Step	0091906539	£4.99
☐ The Bach Remedies Workbook	0091906520	£12.99
☐ Dictionary of the Bach Flower Remedies	0091906490	£4.99

FREE POST AND PACKING
Overseas customers allow £2.00 per paperback

ORDER:

By phone: 01624 677237

By post: Random House Books
c/o Bookpost
PO Box 29
Douglas
Isle of Man, IM99 1BQ

By fax: 01624 670923

By email: bookshop@enterprise.net

Cheques (payable to Bookpost) and credit cards accepted

The prices shown above are correct at time of going to press. However, the publishers reserve the right to increase prices on covers from those previously advertised, without further notice.

Allow 28 days for delivery.

When placing your order, please mention if you do not wish to receive any additional information.

www.randomhouse.co.uk